Wanna Play Yoga?

Create a "Fun"-tastic Kids Yoga Class
in Your Authentic Voice!

Stacey Pinke

Illustrations by Maria Gronowska

ISBN: 978-1-4834-9511-8 (sc)
ISBN: 978-1-4834-9510-1 (e)

Library of Congress Control Number: 2018914767

Because of the dynamic nature of the Internet, any web addresses or links contained in this book may have changed since publication and may no longer be valid. The views expressed in this work are solely those of the author and do not necessarily reflect the views of the publisher, and the publisher hereby disclaims any responsibility for them.

This book is a work of non-fiction. Unless otherwise noted, the author and the publisher make no explicit guarantees as to the accuracy of the information contained in this book and in some cases, names of people and places have been altered to protect their privacy.

Any people depicted in stock imagery provided by Getty Images are models, and such images are being used for illustrative purposes only.
Certain stock imagery © Getty Images.

Lulu Publishing Services rev. date: 10/31/2020

Dedication

I dedicate this book to my mom and dad, my husband Glenn and Debby Kaminsky, Founder of the Newark Yoga Movement.

My mom always told me I have a way with words. She wanted me to share my thoughts with others because she found my energy to be magical, and uplifting. I dedicate this book to my mom who encouraged me to write. I love you always.

I also dedicate this book to my dad, who has instilled in me a great love for adventure. Writing and publishing my first book has been a big adventure! I love you, Dad.

Glenn, thank you for going on this wonderful yoga journey with me. I love how yoga has enriched our lives.

The four years I've worked for the Newark Yoga Movement have been endlessly rewarding. Over the years, Debby suggested I write a book on how to teach yoga classes to children. Finally, the time is right, and here it is. Thanks, Debby, for your encouragement, the work, and your friendship. I love what I do, and I'm so grateful to share in this journey with you!

Wanna Play Yoga?

Create a "Fun"-tastic Kids Yoga Class
in Your Authentic Voice!

PART II

PART III

Foreword

Children are not little adults—neither physiologically nor psychologically. Teaching yoga to children is, as one might expect, not simply replicating content and delivery that one would use in teaching an adult class. Yoga is both a science and a philosophy, but its teaching is an art and its capable practitioner knows that to make a yoga practice accessible to toddlers, children, and young adults, a special approach is needed. Grown-ups can tolerate an hour (or more) long asana sequence, but sixty minutes of uninterrupted direction following is a lot to ask of little yogis.

Indeed, such an effort is destined to fail when one considers, as the developmental psychologist Jan Piaget pointed out, that the older we get, the faster time passes. Conversely, time seems to last much longer for children; for example, for a five-year-old summer seems to stretch on forever, but it goes quite quickly for a fifty-year-old adult. Put in other words, what is to you or me a mere sixty minutes, and perceived as such, is perceived as four or five hours to a young child.

A practical understanding of this difference in time perception, a knowledge of age-appropriate yoga pose sequencing, of child development, and of positive communication techniques is necessary to succeed as a children's yoga teacher.

When yoga teachers construct purposeful lesson plans for children, they consider appropriate poses taught in a sensible order as well as their ability to engage the youngster's body and mind. Opening with a seated centering may work well for adult practitioners, but little folk often need a warm-up game or activity to get themselves grounded and in a peaceful, receptive frame of mind. To keep kids interested, asana sequences need to be broken up with relevant games, stories, and songs. Little imaginations need to be captivated. Swing your arms like Ganesh swinging his trunk, clearing away all the trees in the forest from his way and throwing out of his path every obstacle!

Stacey Pinke is an experienced yoga teacher and consulting nutritionist/dietician who holds much passion and love for what she does and teaches from a place of great compassion, an incisive intellect, and a deep and practical knowledge.

Wanna Play Yoga? is packed with tried and tested ideas for teaching yoga to kids: a perfect go-to book for yoga class suggestions, with material that is well-structured and practical, and clearly and concisely written in a very readable, charming style. Stacey integrates yoga instruction, storytelling, role-playing, and imaginative visualizations to teach healthy living in mind and body, conscious awareness, self-confidence, focus and concentration, balance, self-discipline, and kindness.

Wanna Play Yoga? is the book that I would want to read—thoroughly—before I taught my first children's yoga class. I regard it as an indispensable tool for the newly minted teacher of yoga to children as well as an invaluable resource for the experienced veteran. The sample classes alone are worth the price of the entire book.

William A. Courson, Ayur.D
Dean for Academic Affairs,
Sai Ayurvedic College
Dean of Students, Bodhananda Vedic Institute School of Ayurveda

Montclair, New Jersey
January 16, 2018

Acknowledgments

There are so many people I'd like to thank because so many have either knowingly or unknowingly encouraged me to write this book and helped me along the way. I have done my best to give credit where credit is due. Any omission is simply an oversight, not a slight.

First, I'd like to thank all the yoga instructors who have guided me. Thank you, Claire Diab, owner and founder of the American Yoga Academy, with whom I did my very first yoga teacher training. I want to also give a special thanks to Jen Gold Schulman, who was the very first yoga instructor to guide me on my path. You are a very special, kind soul. Thank you, Agnes Tengerdy-Krauser, for being a magnificent light and a wonderful friend. Cate Baily, Savitri, Betsy Davis, Daniele Jarman, Emma Magenta, Sarah Bodnar and Christina Helms —thanks to all of you for creating beautiful yoga communities in which I enjoy amazing yoga classes! Thank you, Debby Kaminsky, for offering me opportunities to teach yoga to the children in the city of Newark, New Jersey. I have loved guiding the children toward inner peace.

Thank you to my children, my loving husband, and my dear friend Irma, who have all encouraged me to write. Not all my ideas are my own. There's no sense in reinventing the wheel. I give a lot of credit and acknowledgment to the teachers I've come to know and respect: Shari Vilchez-Blatt of Karma Kids Yoga, Cheryl Crawford from Grounded Kids Yoga, Christine McArdle-Oquendo of Om Shree Om, Chara Rodriguera of Sol Path Yoga and Jodi Golda Komitor, founder of Next Generation Yoga. I love the creativity and enthusiasm all of you bring to the profession. With a big heart, I thank *you*!

I want to give heartfelt thanks to Sharon Manner, founder of Ashrams for Autism, who has offered me so many useful insights in guiding children on the autistic spectrum through yoga classes. The Samadhi Sun training you provided was exceptional!

I want to express tremendous gratitude for the shaman I saw in Guatemala at Lake Atitlan at Villa Sumaya.[1] He described my energy as magical and encouraged me to express myself with my hands, either by writing or practicing Reiki. I took his words to heart.

---

[1] http://villasumaya.com. I went on a yoga retreat here, and a shaman did a Mayan reading on me. I had a fabulous experience!

Thank you, Maria, for sharing your amazing talent by illustrating this book. Thank you to Carley, who suggested that Maria illustrate this book. Thank you, Glenn, for helping with the editing.

Thank you, Maureen Murray. Your guidance has been greatly appreciated.

Thank you, Sarah Bodnar of Drishti Design. Your help has been invaluable to me.

Thank you, Savitri, Cate Baily, and Kathryn Livingston for your support, guidance, friendship and yoga.

Thank you, William Courson. Without your guidance this book would have never been published.

With the deepest gratitude to all of you, I have written this book.

Introduction

As a Registered Dietitian and yoga instructor, I've come to realize that positive change starts with a yoga practice because yoga inspires people to take better care of themselves. That desire for improved self-care can translate into improved physical health, mental clarity, better focus, and higher grades for kids who encounter a great deal of stress and pressure to excel in school today.

I include in my classes and in this book yoga *asanas* (poses), breathing, chanting (age and school appropriate), and dharma talks that are age-appropriate life philosophy and self-empowerment skills. Talking to the kids about topics that really matter in a relatable way is what makes my classes so special. If there is no illustration for a pose mentioned in this book, *Yoga Journal* has a reputable website with images.

I wrote this book to inspire kids' yoga instructors to create new classes and to allow those who are curious about teaching to explore the process of creating a class. The dharma chapters are written for instructors to consider as they create a class for children. The chakra chapters briefly explain the chakras to people who are new to teaching yoga to kids. I offer topic ideas for classes and step-by-step sample classes. I hope this book generates new class ideas, confidence, and enthusiasm to teach.

There are many reasons I love working with children. They are so spontaneous and honest. Sometimes while guiding a class, I'll look out into a student's eyes to realize he or she is really getting what I'm saying. I see the light in that child, which is the same as the light in me. At Newark Yoga Movement[2], we end each class by saying, "I see the good in you. You see the good in me. We see the good in each other. *Namaste*." I love these words. It's my hope that over time the children absorb their meaning into their being and their lives. It's the remembrance that there is good in all of us.

I bow to each of you: the parents, teachers, and fellow yoga instructors who take the time to read this book and continue to share your wisdom with children and others.

---

[2] Newarkyogamovement.org

Part I

Chapter 1

Benefits of Yoga for Kids

The benefits of yoga are numerous. Yet, I'm only highlighting a few here.

With a regular yoga practice, sleep quality and digestion may improve, and anxiety abates.

Yoga increases creativity and imagination. Young children, ages five to seven, generally love to make up their own poses and dance. Given these opportunities of free expression, their imagination soars. Through chanting, *pranayama* (breathing), and meditation, students may achieve mental clarity and a quiet mind. In this quiet space, they can hear their intuitive thoughts and creative ideas.

Yoga improves focus and concentration as well as a child's self-esteem. Nailing a pose after working on it for months is cause for celebration. This sense of accomplishment will carry over off the mat as well.

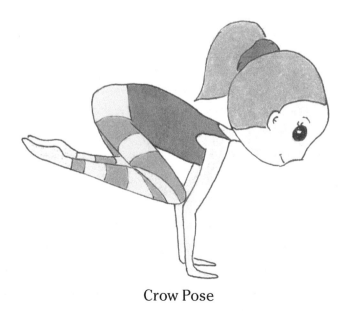

Crow Pose

After months of practice, Jane finally comes into crow pose for two seconds. Admittedly, that is not much time, yet it's an accomplishment to be celebrated. The first time anyone comes into an arm balance, there's a moment of realization. Typically, the practitioner then falters and falls. She has left the awareness of the body and entered the excitement of the mind. This disconnect from the body causes the fall. The fact, though, is that she did it! The body has muscle memory. The next time she can work on holding the pose for a longer time. When Jane has a class project to complete, she will remember how she worked at crow pose and approach the project with the same focus and determination.

The benefits of yoga are more than those mentioned here. My yoga practice has been filled with self-discovery and healing. To understand the benefits, I encourage you, the reader, to explore your yoga practice with curiosity and wonder. Then, let the journey begin.

Chapter 2

Dharma, Yamas, and Niyamas—
What Am I Saying?

Dharma is loosely defined as one's character. My dharma talks touch upon approaches to life and its challenges. The topics include: gratitude, body awareness, mindfulness, letting go, trust, balance, nonattachment, respect, truth, cleanliness, and focus. These dharma talks are engaging because I approach these topics from angles that relate to children.

The *yamas* are ethical standards that focus on the individual and how he/she relates to the surrounding environment. There are five of them: *ahimsa, satya, asteya, brahmacharya,* and *aparigraha*. Ahimsa is nonviolence. Satya is truth. Asteya is not stealing or being respectful. Brahmacharya means balance. Aparigraha is nonattachment to outcomes or going with the flow.

The *niyamas* have to do with self-discipline, introspection, and taking care of oneself. There are five niyamas: *saucha, santosha, tapas, svadhyaya,* and *ishvara pranidhana*. Saucha is cleanliness. Santosha is contentment. Tapas is focus. Svadhyaya is the study of yourself or introspection. Ishvara pradidhana is trust or seeing the bigger picture.

My dharma talks mimic the yamas and niyamas, which are the codes of ethics by which we live. For example, incorporating an attitude of gratitude helps a child have a more positive outlook on life. Gratitude is part of the *niyama santosha*, which means contentment. Ultimately, it is my hope that the reader will be motivated to use my talks and create their own by using the tools and exercises in this book. Dharma talks serve to build a student's character.[3] I think it is important to instill ethical values while teaching a fun and creative class to kids. By offering dharma talks in a yoga class, a child will ultimately learn that wisdom, love, courage and happiness all reside in the body.

---

[3] Chara offers a yoga program called Sol Path Yoga which is based on the yamas and niyamas and has greatly influenced how I practice and teach yoga.

Chapter 3

Gratitude

The practice of gratitude is to appreciate what you have.

"Imagine how you would feel if, when you awoke, you decided to make note of all objects and events for which you are grateful." A yoga instructor said these words to me, and an attitude of gratitude has spun my world into a beautiful place of my own design.

Gratitude for objects, events, and circumstances, both big and small, can help children overcome challenges and stress in their lives.

When discussing gratitude, I may express the following ideas as the students are exploring a pose or the breath. Even during a very challenging moment, they can feel *gratitude for being alive and breathing*.

> What does it mean to be thankful or to appreciate? How does it feel? Imagine what it would be like to wake up and simply notice, all day long, all the things for which you are grateful. Can you only be grateful for happy things? No, you can learn to appreciate hard days and challenges too because they enable you to grow stronger. You can embrace these opportunities to learn. This challenge was created because it was the perfect learning opportunity for you. Without this mistake or upsetting time, maybe you wouldn't have faced a situation in which you ultimately learned a valuable lesson.

Sometimes I reflect on challenges I have overcome and marvel at the universe for creating this perfect healing or learning opportunity for me. I explain these concepts to children and often share a personal story with them, to illustrate my point. As the instructor telling my story, it is important to make the story relatable to the children. I do not want to go on about me or give unnecessary details.

One year, on the first day of January, I was skiing in Colorado with my family. My eight-year-old daughter asked me to race with her down the mountain. I figured, "Why not?" Off I went down the mountain without a care in the world. Soon after beginning the race, I realized I was going too fast. While I tried to slow down, conditions were icy, and I was not successful at stopping. I thought, *It's no big deal. I'll just crash into the mesh netting at the end of the slope.* I was in a fantastic mood, excited for the upcoming year. Nothing was going to get me down.

So I thought. I crashed, landing hard on the snow. Since the ski did not release, my left leg twisted, and I badly injured my knee, which took nine months to heal. During this time, my knee healed and my relationship with my family improved too. I learned that I can rely on family members to help me. It's hard for me to receive help from others and this situation gave me a chance to experience support and feel loved. I'm grateful for all that happened.

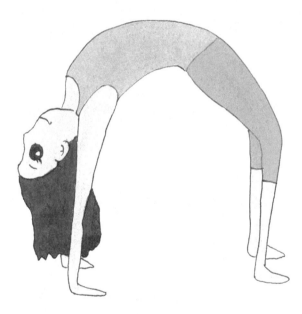

Wheel Pose

Heart-opening poses such as wheel, bridge, and cobra are good to practice during a yoga class with a dharma talk on gratitude.

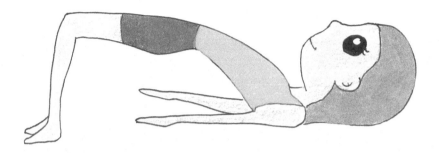

Bridge Pose

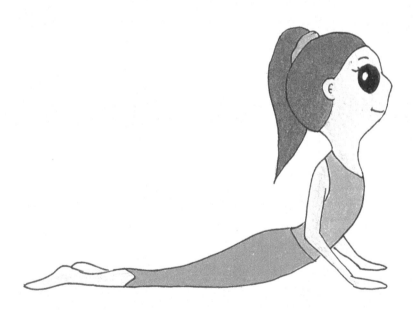

Cobra Pose

In all three poses, the student breathes in and out with the awareness on the heart center. The shoulder blades hug the back, space is created between the shoulder and the ears, and the chest or heart lifts.

Chapter 4
Body Awareness

Body awareness refers to the physical body. How does the body move? How does it appear in the mirror? What are the sensations inside the body?

As the reader of this book, please think about the following, and maybe you'll want to share these thoughts with your yoga students as well.

> You spend your whole life with yourself. There is no greater gift than learning about yourself because the better you understand yourself, the better you can help yourself. You can be your own best friend!

> During the day, you spend so much time focused on the outside world which can be overstimulating. The gift of this practice is to bring the awareness inward. If you are tired, sleep. If you are upset, ask yourself what you need to find happiness. Sometimes you find a peaceful part of you; worries and concerns seem to melt away. By looking inside, you will find answers that will better guide your actions.

As you, the instructor, read the following paragraph, think of an adult example in which you move without awareness. Perhaps you toss your keys on a table and then forget where you've placed them. I use the school hallway and the backpack as examples, to make the concept relatable to children.

> Do you hurry along, bumping into people in the hallway or throwing the backpack down without any regard to where it lands? This happens to everyone at times. Yet you can move more slowly, paying attention to how your body moves through space.

How do you move the body with awareness? Moving slowly is part of the answer; the other part is the breath. The breath is the bridge between the mind and the body. Breathing, in deeply and out fully, quiets the mind and brings awareness into the rest of the body.

Here I show how to guide the children in linking the breath to the movements in washing machine pose[4,] and water wheel. The breath pattern for washing machine pose is through the nose but I suggest open-mouthed breathing when a child has a cold. For children ages three to five, I suggest to breathe in through the nose and out through the mouth as that breath pattern best mimics the sounds of a washing machine. My washing machine pose is different from others in that the arms are in goal post shapes and the fingers are in fists.

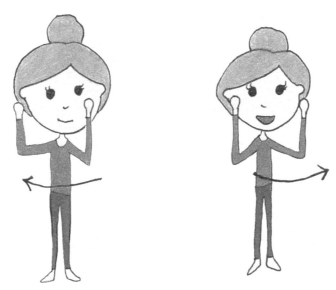

Washing Machine Pose

With arms out to the side, like goal posts, keep your feet firmly planted on the ground. Breathe in through the nose as your belly, chest, and head turn one way. Exhale

---

[4] Many kids' yoga programs offer a variation of washing machine pose and breath. www.groundedkids.com, www.karmakidsyoga.com, www.nextgenerationyoga.com

through the nose or mouth as your belly, chest, and head turn the other way. Repeat and listen. The breathing pattern will sound like the sounds a washing machine makes.

Another excellent combination of asana and breath is linking the pose water wheel to the breath. Water wheel is a high lunge. High lunge is a warrior I with the back heel up and the toes facing forward.

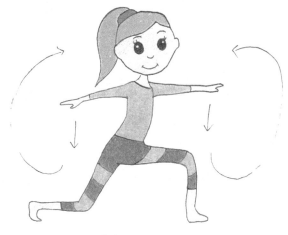

Water Wheel

Breathe in slowly. Your breath is at its fullest when your arms are high. Exhale slowly. Your body is empty of the breath when your arms are down. Let the breath carry you through the movement.

I guide the students into arm circles while making these connections to the breath. At first the movement is simple, and then the children are surprised by how tiring the exercise is.

Exhale when you bend the back knee and lower the back leg and arms. Inhale when you straighten the back leg and raise the arms.

A more advanced practice for the children in fourth grade and up is to try to keep the entire body still except for the back leg and arms. There's often another level to make a pose challenging! The children often express surprise as they attempt this and succeed!

Chapter 5

Mindfulness

Mindfulness, as I describe it to children, is the act of being aware of one's thoughts without criticism. Children can be the witness to the mind, observing the thoughts without judgment. They do not need to know if the thoughts are good or bad.

I invite the reader to consider the following. Whether you're practicing yoga or just living life, you always can bring awareness back to the breath. By focusing on the breath, you can calm the mind. Imagine your thoughts as balloons. Let them float by. Only if you like a thought should you hold onto it. In this way, you are practicing mindfulness and purposefully choosing a positive thought.

I call this the balloon breath meditation.

> Notice the clear blue sky. One balloon, then several appear. Which color or colors are they? *Pause.* Which shapes? *Pause.* Imagine each balloon holds a thought. Watch them drift, float, and swirl. If you do not like the thought, watch the balloon float up and away. Now find a balloon that contains a thought you do like. Imagine you can reach up and pull on a string to draw the balloon down. Carry it with you throughout your day.

> The two following breathing meditations illustrate how to practice mindfulness.

> To achieve greater stillness, place your hands on your abdomen or stomach. Breathe in and imagine your stomach swelling like a balloon. Breathe out. Feel your stomach deflating or shrinking as a balloon would.

> Or notice how thoughts are like waves. They roll in and they roll out. Be a witness to the mind. Watch the waves or the thoughts. Witness the breath ebb and flow in and out of the body.

Is there a space between the thoughts? The practice of mindfulness creates a space between the thoughts, just like there is space between each thought balloon, or each wave cresting.

Another aspect of awareness or mindfulness is words and how they influence the body.

Let's say I have a bowl of water. Let's imagine the water is the world around me, the community in which I live. I also have salt. Let's imagine the salt is the words I choose to use. I can do a demonstration in which I pour the salt into the bowl of water. After I pour the salt in, can I take it out? No, of course, I cannot.[5]

That is the point. When you speak negative, hurtful words, you cannot take them back. The listener feels the pain of the hurtful words.

On the other hand, positive words are uplifting. For example, I feel cheerful when I speak optimistically. Here's a fun exercise that you can do with the kids.

With your arms outstretched, please think of something sad. A friend will try to press your arms down, and it will be relatively easy for him or her to do that. Stretch the arms out in a T-shape again, this time thinking of a happy time. Your friend will attempt to push your arms down again, unsuccessfully.

Happy thinking is powerful![6]

Think about a compliment you have received and notice how the energy changes in the body. What happens to your muscles? Does a smile form on your face?

Have you, the reader, explored these exercises? If not, please do.

---

[5] Peggy Jenkins, "Chapter 11: Watch Your Words," *Nurturing Spirituality in Children: Simple Hands-on Activities.* (Hillsboro, OR: Beyond Words Pub., 1995), 22-23. I am paraphrasing a demonstration found in this book.
[6] Karma Kids Yoga has a similar game called "The Power of Positive Thinking." I discovered this game during the Karma Kids Teen Yoga Teacher Training. Visit Karmakidsyoga.com for more information.

I'd like to emphasize that the practice of mindfulness also applies to a bad mood. I invite the reader to think of a time you were in a bad mood. Observe the sensations of the emotion while observing your breath. As the breath moves in and out of the body, you will notice that the emotions move too. Like a wave, an emotion rolls in and out repeatedly and eventually recedes. These feelings come from the heart. A feeling simply wants to be felt. Once you feel it, you understand yourself better and the intensity of the feeling subsides. It takes courage to let yourself simply feel a bad, sad, or angry feeling. It's hard because when we experience these strong feelings, we want to act. The mind labels the feeling and often thinks up an action. If there is no observation or mindfulness, the body may simply act on the thought. Mindfulness creates a pause between the thought and the action.

Rather than judge thoughts, students can choose. It's up to them to choose positive or negative thoughts to guide their actions. I sometimes have students hold poses such as high lunge, warrior I, or warrior II.

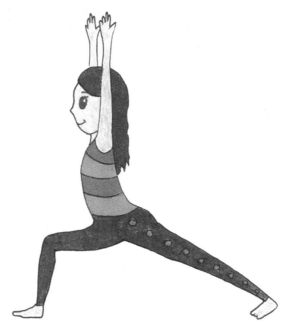

Warrior 1

While holding the pose, do the students focus on the pain of the muscle burning, or do they focus on the gratitude for their strong bodies? This practice combines mindfulness with *santosha* or gratitude.

The more experienced the teacher and student become, the easier it is to shift thoughts to more positive ones. If a student holds a warrior pose, muscles may hurt. You, as the teacher, can suggest that the student shift attention to a part of the body that feels calm or strong. You can suggest the student notice serenity in the heart or strength of the legs. In short, the student can choose a positive, uplifting thought by changing focus.

Chapter 6
Letting Go

When discussing the topic of letting go with children, I like to focus on the uplifting feeling achieved by the act of letting go. Notice if the following idea resonates with you and decide if you would like to share this with children in your class.

> Have you ever had a thought, one that upsets you, and it keeps repeating? Let's explore how to break the cycle. The mind is a thought-generating organ. Observe the thoughts.

Now I'd like the reader to consider this. What is the purpose of anger or sadness? When you feel an intense emotion, is it easier to react or act calmly? Consider your own response when you have a challenging situation. Your honest self-evaluation will help you have more compassion for your students. My point is this. It is easy to react but preferable to go slowly.

Some thoughts are associated with a feeling. The feeling provides you with valuable information about yourself. Once you have this information, you can act in a life-affirming way.

The benefit of letting go is that the old stories of the mind no longer make the student feel down.

I offer a class based on the story of the farmer and the donkey. I put yoga poses to the story, and it has a moral:

> There is a farmer who does not like the donkey on his farm. It is morning.

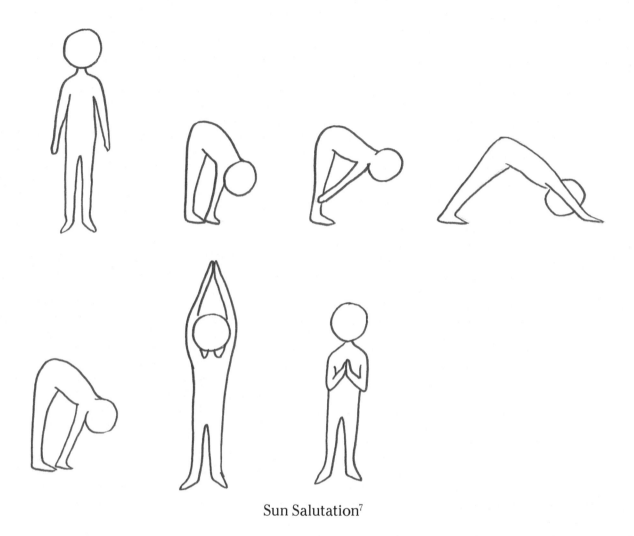

Sun Salutation[7]

He is happy because the sun is shining. He does a sun salutation as a way to say thanks for the day. He hears the donkey making a lot of noise. When he walks back to the prairie, he notices that the donkey has fallen into a hole. He walks to his shed and reaches up for the shovel. (Stretch up for the shovel.)

---

[7] This is my abridged version of sun salutation. For a more complete version of sun salutations, please visit Yoga Journal's website www.yogajournal.com.

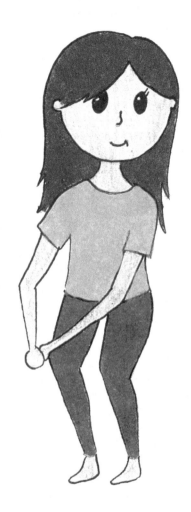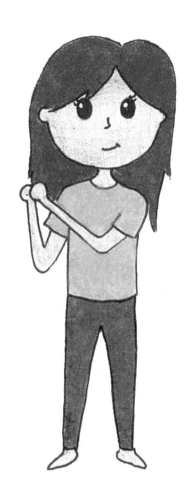

Shovel

He digs a hole next to the one with the donkey (digging motion with bent knees, tossing "dirt" over the shoulder). Because he doesn't like the donkey, he wants to bury him alive. Is that nice? *Discussion.* I offer a series of poses as the donkey trying to shake off the dirt.

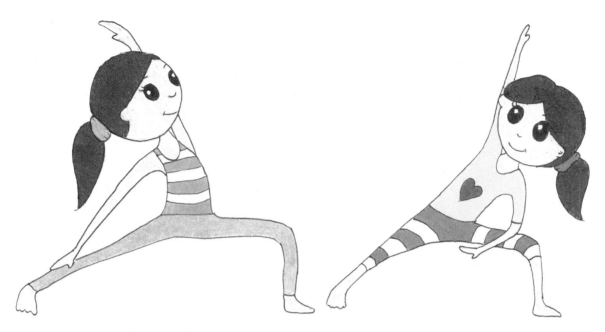

Peaceful Warrior

Side Angle Stretch

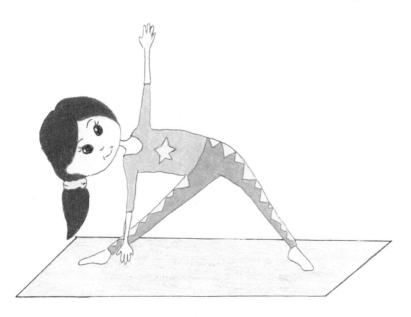

Triangle Pose

Water wheel, peaceful warrior, side angle stretch, triangle. Do these poses on both sides. When you are done, there is a big mound of dirt next to the donkey. He climbs over the dirt and out of the hole. The moral is that when someone is nasty to you, you can shake it off and turn something negative into something positive.

The author of this story is unknown.

Chapter 7
Trust

The topic of trust applies to trusting yourself and life. The niyama *ishvara pranidhana*, which is the practice of trusting or seeing the bigger picture, is most like this dharma talk on trust.

Sometimes you are undecided, and you simply need to be in that space of indecision. You need to trust that you are exactly where you need to be and the experience you are having is the one that will be your best teacher. It's hardest to trust when you are going through a difficult time. Yet, that is most when you need to trust and stick with the process.

> Think of a time of indecision. Two choices pull you in either direction. The mind wants to rush to decide. What are the feelings in the body? Tight stomach? Tense shoulders?

> Think of a time you felt angry. What does the anger feel like? Do you have vibrations in the arms? Does the anger stop you from sleeping well?

Riding the waves of uncertainty or anger is not easy. It's a practice. Trust that this moment presented itself to teach you something valuable.

The world loves to challenge you. If you trust the process, solutions unfold. That is the beauty of simply trusting rather than forcefully trying to control each situation.

When going through a hard time, you might want to press the fast-forward button to avoid facing the hardship, as if that were possible! Especially during moments like this, it's important to realize that you are always exactly where you need to be. There's a valuable lesson to be learned from every situation, challenge, or obstacle. Certainly, it may feel as if a situation is wrong, but therein lies the opportunity to learn. From my biggest mistakes, I've learned my greatest lessons. That's the beauty of trusting that you're right where you need to be. The trust gives you serenity to go with the currents of change or find a way through or around resistance. If you trust in this moment, you surrender to what is. It doesn't mean you give up. Rather, you accept what is.

Here is a suggestion of sequences I may offer in my children's yoga classes:

I like to offer stretching frog pose as a warmup. Then I offer eagle pose, eagle taking flight, funky tree, and chair pose.

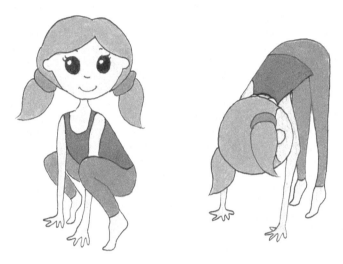

Stretching Frog Pose

To stretch like a frog[8], begin in a squat. Place your hands in front of your toes, flat on the ground. Lift the hips, and the hands stay on the ground. Lower your hips, and lift your beautiful faces. Notice your breath pattern as you enjoy this stretch.

---

[8] Grounded Kids Yoga has a similar pose called Get Up. Please check out www.Groundedkids.com.

I offer stretching frog pose a few times depending on the endurance of the class. We stop when they are tired. This frog pose stretches, strengthens, energizes and calms the body.

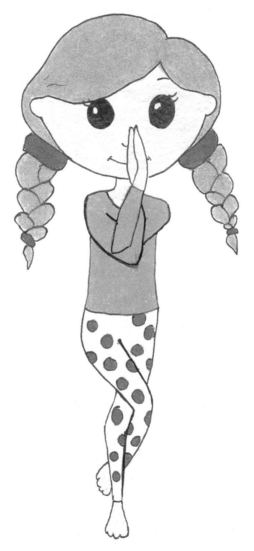

Eagle Pose

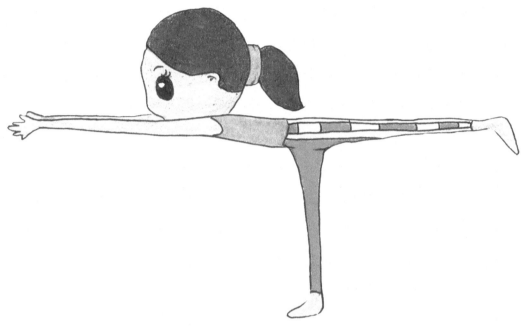

Warrior III Pose

Eagles have keen vision and a large perspective of the view below because they are up high. Eagles are very strong too. Be like an eagle. See all and then decide the next move. Eagle taking flight is a warrior III pose. It requires an element of trust. Bring your heart forward as you press your heel back on an imaginary wall.

Sometimes you feel isolated. The illusion is that you are alone. In truth, you are never alone, and by trusting this, you can feel more peaceful. Be like the eagle who sees the big picture. Notice all the people in this room with you. Think about all the people in this town who are part of your community.

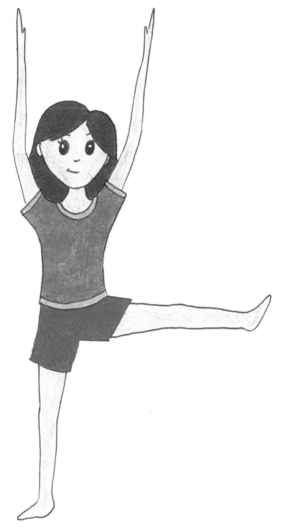

Funky Tree

Funky tree is tree pose in which you straighten the bent leg and bring it out to the side like a branch. This pose requires strength, focus, and balance.

We've already discussed the challenges of water wheel (see Chapter 4 Body Awareness).

Practice poses that the students can hold for long periods, such as warrior poses, repetitive water wheels and chair pose. The students' muscles will get tired. The mind will say it wants to stop. By focusing on the breath and a positive thought, the student will learn to persevere in the face of a challenge. With practice, a student will learn that a challenging situation is an opportunity for personal growth.

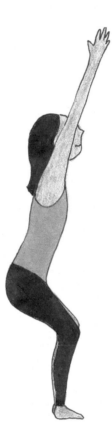

Chair Pose

Chapter 8

Balance

I love teaching classes focused on balance. The topic of balance is a pairing of opposites: rest/ activity, receive/give, left/right, noisy/quiet, inhalation/exhalation, and flexibility/strength.

The yama of *brahmacharya*, which translates as self-control, means to live in moderation or balance. In all ways, your body wants balance. Another word for balance is homeostasis. If a food is salty and/or dry, you want liquids.

Focus on the breath and notice how it ebbs and flows between inhalation and exhalation. Even if you hold your breath, you will need to breathe out eventually.

Nadi shodhana breathing, also called alternate nostril breath, is a breathing exercise that balances the two hemispheres of the brain so that your brain works at its very best. For a description of this breathing exercise, see Chapter 16, section Breath.

Being in balance helps you feel whole, complete, and free to be who you are. Does that mean you are free to do whatever you want, whenever you want? What if every day were a long and relaxing day? Initially, it may be great! Think of the long days of summer. However, may you feel bored as the months go by? The opposite of relaxation is being busy. To enjoy relaxation, it needs to be paired or balanced with busyness.

Some yoga poses both strengthen and stretch the body. If the bottom half of our body is firmly grounded, rooted, and stable on the earth, then the upper half has freedom and flexibility. If you only stretched, you would be very flexible, but you would lack muscle tone for strength. Your body needs both flexibility and strength to be healthy. Tree, warrior, and side plank poses are examples.

Chapter 9
Nonattachment

Aparigraha is the Sanskrit word that means non-attachment. You are in the moment, going with the flow. It's the experience that matters, not the outcome. It's what you learn along the way that counts, not the results.

During the yoga asana practice, let go of the concept of how you think the pose is supposed to look. Focus on how it feels to be in the pose. Be curious about the experience. Work on the pose from the inside out.

You want your version of eagle pose to look like the instructor's, but it doesn't. Accept that your arms or legs don't double cross or that your palms don't meet. Shift your focus to the subtle movements of the breath. The mind quiets. Enjoy the pose the way it is.

You know what you want and then you need to accept what is. It's great to have goals, but what happens when life doesn't give you what you want? You focus and work hard, yet you may only get a C or a D, not an A on the exam. You want to go to the water park, but it rains, and plans get canceled. It is normal to feel disappointed when you don't get the desired result. Yet if you remain calm when it rains, maybe you can run with friends in the rain or stay inside, cozy, with a good book or movie. Non-attachment to outcome enables you to learn from the experience and remain comfortable with what is.

To practice non-attachment, you can have the children switch partners while practicing partner poses.

Explore the idea that you are not your belongings. You have value without them. When you attach emotionally to your possessions, you think they define who you are. They do not. You are often taught to share what you have: a toy, a pencil, or food. It's great to share, and I think that the biggest gift you can give someone is simply sharing time together.

Here's a meditation:

> Let's be like a picnic blanket. Okay, you may be wondering what that means. A picnic blanket is placed on the dirt or grass in a park. When kids run over it or people walk around, dirt may be kicked up onto the blanket. Food crumbs land on it. Perhaps it begins to rain and/or the wind blows. The point is that no matter what contacts the blanket, the blanket rejects nothing. Neither does it hold onto things. A beverage may spill and still the blanket lets the spill rest until someone wipes it up. It doesn't fret or try to control who or what goes on it. Let's be like that blanket. Let's be neutral. Whatever is, it is just this way for this moment. Please just let it be, without judgment. With this neutral mind, you can go with the flow.

If you feel, "No way, I cannot deal with this," then the practice would be to simply observe that this is where your thoughts are. Accept what is and go from there.

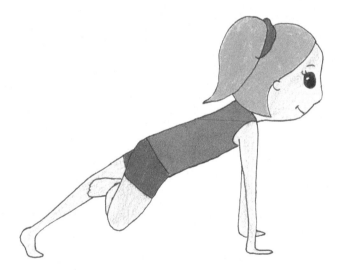

I also like to practice aparigraha as doing tree pose in plank pose. In tree pose, the student stands on one leg, bends the other knee, and places the opposing foot on the ankle, calf, or upper thigh of the standing leg. Offering tree in plank pose means the student would be on curled toes and palm with one knee bent and the foot on the ankle, calf, or thigh of the straight leg. Are you attached to tree in one particular plane?

Chapter 10
Respect

Respect is a broad topic because there are different ways, we respect ourselves and others. Being kind to yourself is one form of respect. It includes exercising in moderation, eating healthfully, and handling our bodies and minds in an unharmful way. The words we speak affect our mental health. Kindness keeps the mind happy and the body healthy. Being respectful to others means being non-injurious in words and action. Being polite is appropriate, especially when you disagree with what another person says or does.

The yoga instructor may engage the students by asking the following questions.

> What does the word *respect* mean? How do you show yourself respect? How do you show respect to others?

Being kind to yourself means not overextending yourself and giving yourself time alone to relax if that is what you need. It may mean saying no to other people's requests. Saying no does not necessarily mean you are being rude to the person. You are giving yourself time and energy to pursue something you think is exciting. Sometimes you need to say no to someone else, so you can say yes to you. Being respectful to yourself allows you to live your truth. (see Chapter 11: Truth).

Being respectful also means speaking kindly to yourself and others. Please take the kindness challenge:

> Every time you hear a negative thought in your mind, how do you change it to a more positive thought? When a student says, "I can't do this!" I say, "We don't say that in my class. You simply haven't done it yet!" The sentence, "I haven't done it yet," opens the possibility that one day it will happen.

The kindness challenge requires that you notice your negative thoughts and practice changing them to words that are neutral or positive. This practice is described in Chapter 18 How to Practice Yoga Off the Mat.

On the mat, being respectful means being quiet and aware of your body, thoughts, and movements. Showing respect means acknowledging where your boundaries are. Work to your outer edge of comfort, not more than that. Hold a pose so that it feels comfortable or strengthening or gives you a good stretch. A pose should not hurt. It should feel good. To respect your own yoga practice means to appreciate where you are. Honor your body and the messages it gives you. There is no need for your expression of the pose to look like your neighbors'. Simply do what you can and feel good about what you do. If a pose provides too big of a stretch, respect the limitations of your body, and make yourself comfortable.

Being respectful to yourself and others is important because this practice elevates energy toward love and positivity. When people act in a genuine and kind way, each one feels connected and valued. Ultimately, each person makes a meaningful contribution to the group.

Chapter 11
Truth

Satya is the practice of being truthful to yourself and others. *Sat* is the Sanskrit word for truth. It's that quiet voice inside that whispers your truth. When you are speaking your truth, there is no need to shout. You can follow this inner guidance both on and off the mat.

How do you speak your truth with integrity? You speak calmly and with confidence. Follow your heart and pursue your own interests in a way that leaves you feeling happy and satisfied. Speaking and living your truth are practices that enhance self-respect. (See Chapter 10: Respect).

Spend time with friends who make you feel good about yourself. This is a big one. It drains your energy and makes you feel crummy when you hang out with people who are mean or manipulate you. Above all else, be honest with yourself. Be yourself. Share the magic of being you!

A few breathing exercises help to identify truth. Washing machine pose helps clean the clutter from the mind. Bee breath helps silence the mind to hear the quiet truth. Both are described in Chapter 16 in the section Breath. Repeating the Sanskrit words *Sat Nam* also helps to identify the truth. *Nam* translates to *identity*. *Sat Nam* loosely translates to "I am truth. Truth I am." Students can breathe in while thinking the word Sat and breathe out while thinking the word *Nam*. Alternatively, these words, in either English or Sanskrit, can be spoken aloud.

During class, whichever poses are practiced, the focus will be internal. You may suggest to the students to keep their eyes closed to see inside more clearly.

Chapter 12
Cleanliness

Saucha, in Sanskrit, means cleanliness. More specifically, it means taking care of oneself. Eating healthy foods makes you feel energized and happy. Consuming excess sugar and processed sugar would not be part of your saucha practice.

By contrast, fruits and vegetables consumed in the portions that nature intended would be food that promotes saucha. Fruits and vegetables grow on the earth with the aid of water and sunshine. When you eat these foods, you feel the vitality that comes from the sun. Mother Nature, without the assistance of genetic modification, gives you the complete, wholesome package. Fruits and vegetables have the correct amount and proportion of fiber, water, vitamins, minerals, micronutrients, and antioxidants we need.

When holding a pose, if it causes pain, see how you can modify the pose to make your body more comfortable. You can stretch and strengthen in a pose. Part of the practice of *saucha* or cleanliness is to keep the body free of pain.

Twisting poses are an essential part of a class on cleanliness. A participant will wring out toxins by doing washing machine pose and cat stretch.

Some breathing exercises are excellent for cleansing the body. Breath of fire is one of them. To do breath of fire, concentrate on the exhalations. Pump the navel in each time you exhale through the nose. The inhalation through the nose will occur automatically. Nadi Shodhana breath is very cleansing and calming for the mind. Every time you breathe out, you are clearing your body of stress and carbon dioxide. I explain to children in fourth grade and up that people breathe in oxygen and breathe out carbon dioxide. Plants and trees breathe in carbon dioxide through photosynthesis and release oxygen. We need each other. This fun fact can also be mentioned in a class about balance. (See Chapter 8: Balance).

Be sincere and honest in your words. Let the poor, negative, or hostile ones float away as if they are being packaged in thought balloons. Avoid gossiping. This may seem irrelevant to health, yet it has a strong connection to wellness. How do you feel when someone makes comments that aren't nice? You may feel sad or angry. The words hurt. How do you feel when someone says kind words to you and gives you praise? You may feel happy and light.

Mr. Masaru Emoto, a Japanese scientist, did research that showed on a cellular level the vibration of your words affect you. Mr. Masaru conducted scientific experiments in which he froze water crystals. He exposed water to either high-frequency words (positive) or low-frequency words (negative) in the form of written words or music. Heavy metal music, for example, made the crystal look blurry. Vivaldi music made beautiful, well-defined crystals.[9]

---

[9] Masaru Emoto, *The Hidden Messages in Water.* (Hillsboro, OR: Beyond Words Pub., 2004).

Chapter 13

Focus

The practice of focus is to bring your attention to one activity only. The practice is the same as the niyama of *tapas*. Don't give up when there is a challenge; keep focused on the goal. In a pose that strengthens muscles, focus on your breath, and appreciate the strength of your body. You will feel good about yourself as your body gets stronger. When you are faced with a challenge off the yoga mat, concentrate on what you can learn from this experience or focus on possible solutions. You will feel better chipping away at a problem rather than giving up. It doesn't matter how many times you fail; what matters is that you never give up. You only need one success. If you give up, only one thing is for sure. You will never succeed. Don't say, "I can't." Say that you haven't done it yet! Stay focused and positive in your heart and mind. Remember Jane who succeeded in crow pose in Chapter One.

For the student who insists that a pose is very uncomfortable, I offer encouragement. I may say the following when a student is holding a challenging pose, such as a plank.

> Is it hard to hold this pose? Is it impossible or simply a challenge? Keep trying. Think about how strong you are. Tell yourself you can do it.

Here are a few simple suggestions on how to practice focus on and off the mat each day.

- Show up on your yoga mat.
- Attend school.
- Do your homework.

Chapter 14
Energy Centers or Chakras

There are numerous energy centers or chakras in the body, too many to mention. I've listed the seven main ones that run along the spine, in English, starting at the bottom going to the top. *Chakra* is a Sanskrit word that means wheel or center. When the energy centers are open, you will feel uplifting and positive emotions. All the chakras are interconnected. If one is blocked, the energies of the others will be influenced. A color and a sound are associated with each of the seven main chakras. None of the sounds have meaning. Their significance is in the vibration they create in the body. The vibration unblocks the chakra.

There are many approaches to teaching a yoga class based on the chakras. Ask the children how they feel when they see a rainbow. Their answers will be filled with wonder and happiness. Ask the children what their favorite colors are and how they feel when they see those colors. I may explain that the chakras give off energy. *If you rub your hands together and then separate them, you may feel a tingling sensation or energy between the hands.* After a yoga class with a lot of movement, I ask the students to lay down. I hold a metal necklace above the centers of the spine, and the necklace swings in big circles because the chakras are open.[10] The metal conducts the energy. The children get very excited. I do the metal necklace activity with children ages eight to ten. I have had classes on rainbows, energy that you share, a color, and poses that activate a chakra.

Descriptions of the chakras, and suggested poses and activities for each, follow.

---

[10] I first learned of this technique from Christine McArdle-Oquendo of Om Shree Om. www.christinemcardleoquendo.com

Root Chakra

The color of the root center is red. Its origin is at the base of the spine. The sound is lam. The root center is called the *muladhara chakra* in Sanskrit. Its energy is grounding and stabilizing. The element is the earth. Think of trees and plants, which take root in the ground. When this center is blocked, you feel vulnerable or greedy. When your root chakra is open, you feel safe, protected, and loved.

Offering a class with the theme of hiking is perfect to highlight the root chakra. Plants and trees come from the earth. Rain hits the ground. Any standing or kneeling pose can be associated with the root chakra by focusing on where the body contacts the earth. You can discuss worms: what they do and who in the class loves them! Tree pose is excellent for illustrating the connection the student has with the ground.

Imagine roots growing beneath your feet.

Freeze dancing can be a fun activity for the root chakra because when the students freeze, they focus on their connection to the earth. To make the game more challenging, the students can freeze in a yoga pose that you, the instructor, call out.

Sacral Chakra

The color of the sacral center is orange. This chakra is just below the naval. The sound is vam. It's the chakra of creation or creativity. The sound is vam. It's called the *svadhisthana chakra* in Sanskrit. The element is water. Think of how creativity flows like water. When this chakra is out of balance, you may be fearful, out of touch with your feelings, or resistant to change. When it's open, you feel light, free, and creative.

Activities include coloring and dancing because the students express their creativity through drawing and movement. Discussing what a yoga flow is leads to a fun activity in which each student adds a pose to the existing one.

Everyone places their mats as petals of a flower, in a circle. One person does a pose. Everyone does that pose, and then the next person adds a pose. Each person does both poses. The next person in the circle adds a third pose, and all three poses are done by everyone. This pattern continues until everyone has a turn adding a pose. The result is a unique yoga flow sequence during which everyone experiences what it is like to flow from one pose to the next. Kids happen to love this activity!

Solar Plexus Chakra

The color of the solar plexus center is yellow. It's located above the navel. The sound is ram. The solar plexus center is called the *manipura chakra* in Sanskrit. It's the center of self-esteem and confidence and the element is fire. Think of a digestive fire that not only digests food but your thoughts and emotions too, so that you understand yourself better. Have you ever experienced low self-esteem, felt intense anger, or behaved like a perfectionist? Your solar plexus chakra was closed. When this chakra is open, you feel confident and digest food well.

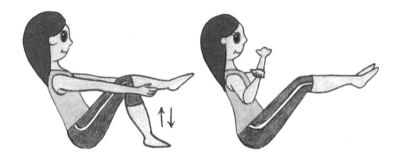

Boat Pose

Activities include singing, meditation and a yoga pose game. Participants may hold boat pose without "sinking." They hold boat pose if they are comfortable and enjoying the ride. Students are instructed to be mindful of the body sensations and to respect the limits of the physical body. The children can meditate by imagining yellow above the navel and observing the physical sensations in that area. Warrior poses, twists, and boat pose stimulate the solar plexus as do singing and meditation.

Heart Chakra

The color of the heart center is green. Sometimes people say the color is pink too. The sound is yum. In Sanskrit, it is called the *anahata chakra*. Its element is air. If you feel lonely, or suffer from heart disease, your heart chakra may be closed. The heart center is the center of compassion and love. This is the chakra that helps us feel connection to others. When the heart chakra is open, blood flows freely and the heart pumps healthfully. You feel happy, loved, and peaceful.

I recommend the following activities to activate the heart chakra. It's useful to say affirmations such as, "I am unique and special" to help a child be centered in love and compassion. I give children paper hearts made of colored construction paper to color, design, or write kind words. Eagle pose and camel pose open the heart chakra.

Throat Chakra

The color of the throat center is blue, and the sound is hum. The throat chakra is the center of communication. In Sanskrit it is called the *vishuddha chakra*. Its element is ether. If you suffer from sinus infections or bronchitis, your throat chakra may be closed. This chakra supplies energy to the thyroid, vocal cords, and lungs. When this energy center is in balance, you can effectively communicate your feelings and needs. You know where your boundaries are.

I recommend the following activities to stimulate the throat chakra. I love to read the book *A Bad Case of Stripes* by David Shannon to illustrate the importance of speaking truthfully. A girl gets very sick because she is too embarrassed to admit her truth, which is that she likes lima beans. A discussion can follow about how it feels to lie. Journaling or coloring after *savasana* (relaxation pose) are good activities to help children explore their truth. Bridge pose and candlestick pose activate the throat chakra.

Brow Chakra

The color of the brow center is indigo. The sound is om, pronounced "aum." It is in the center of the forehead and between the eyebrows. This is the center of intuition, also known as the *third eye*. There is no element for this center. It is governed by light. This chakra supplies energy to the lower brain and the nervous system. Included in this area is the pituitary gland. Nightmares and headaches may mean your brow chakra is closed. Massaging the forehead activates the third eye.

Activities that stimulate this chakra are passive and help quiet the mind. I recommend meditating by looking at a candle and focusing on the breath as it goes in and out of the body. Inviting the children to listen to the quiet around them is a fascinating activity. As the internal chatter of the mind quiets, students tend to notice all the background sounds the environment offers.

Crown Chakra

The color of the crown chakra is purple or white, and the sound is silence. The crown is the top of the head. In Sanskrit it is called the *sahasrara chakra*. Its element is space, and it is very sensitive to light as well. This center may be closed if you are feeling very materialistic. By that I mean, no matter how much you purchase, there is always the next item you want to buy. Or if you are feeling like an intellectual snob, this center may be blocked. The energy from this chakra is about the connection you have with the world around you and the spiritual realm. It's the part of your personality, which taps into higher consciousness and gives you wisdom.

Mandalas are geometric images representing the universe in Hindu and Buddhist symbolism, and they have the power to help focus the mind. Children love to color these mandala images because it is both relaxing and engaging. Mandalas to color can be purchased at a book store or online. Listening to chimes or singing bowls is also very beneficial to achieving a meditative state

Chakras or energy centers govern mental and physical wellness. If one of the chakras is blocked, none of them work well. If one or more is blocked for a prolonged period, illness occurs. Learning how to unblock the chakras is a tool for emotional and physical stability. Ultimately, children will begin to explore ways to self-regulate, calm, and nurture themselves.

Part II

Chapter 15

The Planning Stages

There are many aspects to planning a class. First, I'll discuss the practical matters: location, length of class, time of day, setup and variety of activities for the students. Then, I'll move onto the creative considerations: class ideas and fun facts that impart information in an interesting and imaginative way.

Time, Location and Setup

The location of the class determines the length and the setup. When yoga is offered in the classroom, it typically serves as a break from work, and a class will last ten to twenty minutes. I offer short sessions consisting of breathing techniques, poses, and meditation to increase calm and focus. In the classes with the youngest students, Pre-K or kindergarteners, the students meet on the rug in a designated section of the room. First grade and up, students explore yoga right at their desks. I typically keep chairs and tables where they are to be the least disruptive to the classroom layout. I guide the students through the following short sequence to make sure they have space to move in poses without bumping into objects. If needed, I'll move a student to a more spacious area in the room.

> Please stand in a star pose. Please bring the feet together and swing your arms.
> This is your yoga space.

As an after-school enrichment (ASE), classes are typically offered in a gym or a library. In this environment, an instructor is generally allotted an hour. Allot fifteen minutes for attendance and setup. Plan for a forty-five-minute yoga class. I will configure the mats in a circle or in rows. (View Chapter 16, section Class Arrangement for more details). Sometimes in a library, the floor is carpeted or there is a section with a rug. Both add extra padding when yoga poses are practiced. Still, I prefer to use a mat as it shows where the student's yoga spot is. At some schools, the instructor needs to stay until the parents come to pick up the children. In other schools, a staff member remains with the children until they are picked up.

In a yoga studio, the instructor should plan to be there for an hour. Kids' classes are often scheduled for forty-five minutes. Yet, the instructor needs to set up the mats in a circle or in rows ahead of time. Children are checked in as soon as they enter the studio. They show up early to remove their shoes and stay a few minutes late to put them on. In many cases you will have to bring your own props and you can bring them in a small rolling suitcase. However, some yoga studios cater to children's yoga and provide the necessary props.

A Variety of Activities

When I plan a kid's yoga class, variety is key. Some like to draw. Some like to talk. Others enjoy listening to sound: words, music or a story. Some are captivated by colorful pictures or objects. Many children love to move.

Since some people learn visually, I typically demonstrate poses.

Some people learn by listening. I give short verbal cues to hold their attention.

> Lift arms. Thumbs face back.

This simple cue, "Thumbs face back," achieves hugging the shoulder blades onto the back for support of the spine and midsection.

Hearing music may help children focus on the activity: coloring, writing or doing a few yoga poses in a sequence. Music with soothing lyrics or a peaceful instrumental arrangement may help students feel more centered and tranquil during relaxation pose.

I introduce music when it enhances learning; it cannot distract the student. Sometimes children feel less inhibited to dance when they enjoy the music. Other children are more sensitive to sound, and it may irritate them.

Some people learn by doing and moving. Drawing, writing, creative movement, dancing and linking yoga poses into a flow are great for the student who is restless as well as for the one who is action-oriented.

Activities engage many participants for varying reasons. Picture books with rhyming lyrics are attention grabbers for both the visual and auditory learners. You can also engage the kinesthetic learner, who learns through movement or doing something, by having the student read a passage or answer questions about the illustrations.

It's best to have a lot of activities in a class: yoga poses, games, breathing exercises, readings, coloring, chanting, and meditations to capture the attention of all these young learners. Your classes will be fun and engaging both physically and mentally, stretching and strengthening their physical bodies and expanding their imagination and intellect.

Class Ideas

What gives you inspiration? Maybe it comes from movies, songs, books, or websites. Collect anecdotes from your life. I like to collect quotes. Be creative. The seasons may inspire you with a topic. See where your passions are. Maybe a food or a hobby will give rise to an idea for the class. It sometimes works well to have a playful theme and a dharma talk in the same class. A dharma talk on focus or balance may work nicely with an Olympic-themed class. Here is a list of possible class ideas or themes.

- Visit a country, its people, customs, animals, plants, trees, foods
- Trip to the zoo—which animals do you see there?
- Travel through space
- Hiking
- Olympics: focus on poses that strengthen and stretch. Endurance and flexibility are key. At the end of class, everyone is a winner because everyone has a unique talent or strength.
- Obstacle course
- A special place: What does it look like? What happens there? It could be your special place, or each participant could tell part of a story describing a special place and offering poses to go with it.
- Holidays
- Snow
- Water
- Pause: the space between poses or activity
- Motion verses commotion: motion is fluid. Commotion is chaotic. We want the former because it feels better.

- Peace
- Spring, new beginnings

Three years ago, I was listening to the song "Respect" by Aretha Franklin. Singing and listening to the song, I realized that a dharma talk about respect, along with dancing to this song, would be part of a fun class. My fun facts would be telling the class who Aretha Franklin was and what she accomplished. I'd also teach the children how to spell the word *respect*: r-e–s-p-e-c-t!

I saw a *National Geographic* television show about animals in the Antarctic. That prompted more fun facts:

- The Antarctic or Antarctica is as far down on the map or as far south on the Earth as you can go.
- Antarctica is where the South Pole is.

I'd show the students a picture of an albatross bird.

- It takes the albatross up to ten months to learn how to fly!

Why?

> It takes this long because the bird has very, very large wings. The bird is incredibly clumsy at first. Yet, with all the ups and downs (literally!) along the way, she does not give up, and she does not emotionally beat herself up. While repeatedly approaching the task of learning how to fly, she treats herself with respect. She is patient. If she can be patient with something that may take her ten months to learn, I think, class, that you can be patient learning some yoga poses.

Each student practices patience and respect on the mat while doing yoga and ultimately, learns about himself/herself. Along the way, he/she learns fun facts about the albatross, Antarctica and Aretha Franklin!

Animal Fun Facts

Fun facts are educational information which enables children to learn in a playful way. I've learned many of these fun facts while on African Safaris.

- When zebras are happy, they make the sound, "Bray!" When a zebra is lost, it calls, "Koukoukooroo!" to find its mom.
- When a hippopotamus sunbathes, it turns pink. Blood rushes to the surface of the skin, turning it pink. This pink pigment or color works as a sunscreen for the hippo. If it's a class of children ages eight to ten, I may explain that the word *pigment* is often used to describe the color of the skin.
- Polar bears' fur keeps them warm. Each piece of hair is a tube, like a straw, letting sunlight and warmth pass through.
- The male sea horse carries its young.
- The elephant has 40,000 muscles with 150,000 sections just in his trunk. They are like cylindrical disks that unfurl and collapse. The trunk can twist, spiral, expand, and elongate.
- The male kangaroo carries its young.
- Giraffe's heart weighs about twenty-five pounds and beats sixty-six times per minute when the giraffe is resting. It beats approximately one hundred seventy beats per minute when the giraffe is running.
- The panther species includes lions and leopards. The vocal cords stretch so they can make loud, rough, growling sounds. In the savanna sounds travel further at night. Also, lions and leopards are nocturnal, and they have better vision at night. For all these reasons, lions and leopards hunt at night.
- Animals that are up during the day are called diurnal and include impalas, deer, and waterbuck.

Chapter 16

Putting It All Together

Do What You Love

Often, I am asked, "How do you create a class?" I often include a dharma talk and breath work. Additionally, I put in what I love. This approach makes a class mine. I use my sense of humor, activities I love, and animal fun facts, as mentioned in Chapter 15. I basically include information about anything and everything that is of interest to me.

During my first yoga teacher training I was told to fill a class with what I love. Over the years, I've included Spanish vocabulary, fun facts, favorite songs, and games in my classes.

Here is an enjoyable activity to get you started. On a blank piece of paper, list the things you love. Truly anything can go on the list: people, places, objects, memories, activities, jokes, quotes—to name a few. Don't rush, and the list can be as long as you want. Through self-observation, recognize what you love and add it to the list.

As a kids' yoga instructor, I often need to be spontaneous. Maybe the planned class won't work because the energy of the room does not fit the energy of the class I planned. How do I prepare to be ready for anything?

I try to plan more than I am going to use in a children's yoga class. I'll never know ahead of time what the energy of the room will be and what kind of a day the students have had. It's best to come prepared. It's better to have too much prepared than to have too little. Sometimes I need to completely ditch the class I've planned to simply give the students what I know they need at that moment.

Being able to effectively read class energy is a skill that is mastered with time. Strive for balance in each class. Some class designs are mellower for sure, but you do not want an action-packed class that leaves little or no time for rest.

- If the class is restless or the energy is low, you want to engage them in an uplifting flow followed by something peaceful.
- When a class is very high energy, then you want a more calming class.

Here are some additional thoughts and practices to consider if children are not cooperating. Sometimes the quickest way to have students cooperate is to offer them something fun. Try something silly like dancing. Put on upbeat music and shake out the jitters. Physical activity releases hormones that make people feel more positive and focused.

Yoga is a practice, not a perfect. Kids will not always behave the way you would like. If you notice yourself getting frustrated by their behavior, ask yourself why it is so important that they do what you want. Here is a reminder. This is their class to explore and learn about themselves. It may also be your chance to learn about yourself. Practice letting go by releasing expectations and non-attachment by relinquishing control of the outcome. Practice being present by observing what is currently occurring in the group. Encourage the students to be curious and give them a safe space in which to practice. If students are making noise, incorporate sound, animal noises or words into the yoga practice. If students seem disinterested, let them choose a pose or play the *tingshas*. (See Chapter 16 Putting It All Together, section: Props). By being present, you can make decisions which address their needs.

Breath

The first necessary component of a class is the breath. Breathing is the link between the mind and the body. If I can get a group of children to slow down their breath, I've relaxed them. If I get them to steady their breath, they're focused.

Breathing helps heal the body. Oxygen and nutrients from food are transported through the red blood cells in the arteries to every cell in the body. This circulation of blood, nutrients, and oxygen keeps us alive and healthy. Basically, the more deeply we breathe, the more vibrant we feel. Breathing, or *pranayama*, as it is called in Sanskrit, keeps us performing at our best.

Here are some breathing exercises I enjoy doing with the children. They are bee breath, ribbit, coconuts, bananas, lion's breath, *nadi shodana* or alternate nostril breathing and washing machine breath.[11]

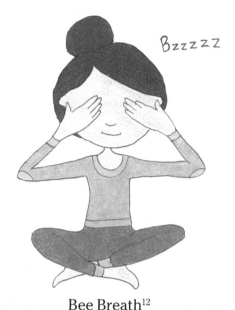

Bee Breath[12]

The bee breath is a very relaxing breathing exercise that incorporates the voice as well. Place the thumbs over the ears and fingers over the eyes. Breathe in, and as you exhale hum "*buzzzz*." You'll hear the vibration within your head. With the eyes and ears closed, your senses are withdrawn from the outside world. You'll feel more peaceful.

---

[11] I absolutely loved the Karma Kids Yoga Teacher Training by Shari Vilchez-Blatt! I learned to put sounds with animal poses including buzzing like a bee, roaring like a lion, ribbiting like a frog and tapping my chest while growling like a gorilla.

[12] Yoga Pretzels by Tara Guber and Leah Kalish. In their version, the eyes and ears are not covered.

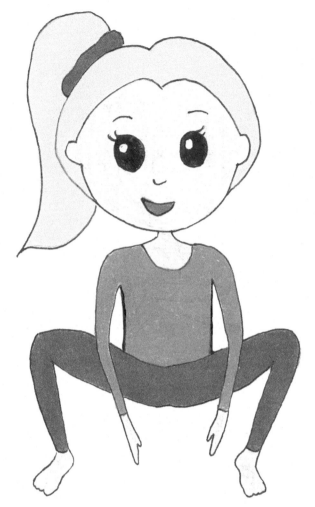

Frog Pose

When the kids explore a frog pose, I may have them repeat the word "ribbit." This frog pose is not the same as the stretching frog pose (see Chapter 7 Trust). This frog is a squat. As the children jump from lily pad to lily pad (or from mat to mat), they say "ribbit" when exhaling. If yoga is given in the classroom, I have "my frogs" jump and say "ribbit" in place.

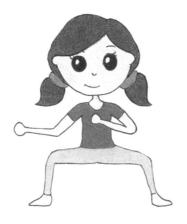

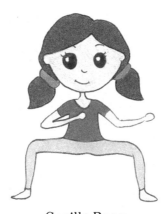

Gorilla Pose

The gorilla eats bananas and coconuts. The children stand in gorilla pose, breathe in, and on the exhalation, say, "Bananaaas," while gently tapping the sternum of the chest. The tapping causes their voice to vibrate. Tapping the sternum also brings about a sense of calm in the body because an acupressure point on the sternum gets activated with the tapping. The breath pattern and tapping can be done while the children say "Coconuuuts!"[13]

_____

[13] Both Shari VIlchez-Blatt of Karma Kids Yoga and Marsha Wenig of YogaKids have the children tap their chest or thymus gland while creating sounds. YogaKids calls this breath Tarzan's Thymus Tap. Karma Kids call it Gorilla Breath. Please check out the work of these two women who have pioneered ways to teach yoga to children.

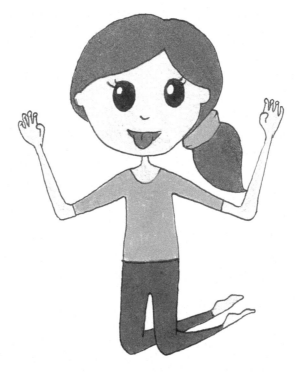

Lion's Breath

For lion's breath, you can either stand or kneel. If you are kneeling, you are only on your knees and shins. The tops of feet are down, or the toes are curled under. Breathe in and take your lion paws out. Imagine that the hands are paws and the fingers are claws. Stick out your tongue and give a quiet roar. Kids love this. I usually do it three times. With this breath, you detoxify your internal organs. When you exhale, press the navel into the abdomen and back.[14, 15]

---

[14] Shari Vilchez-Blatt of Karma Kids Yoga offers lion's pose in Karma Kids Yoga Teacher Training. She encourages her students in lion's pose to roar, whimper or hiss while I say to roar. YogaKids has a similar lion pose in which the "lions" make sounds with each letter of the alphabet. Please feel free to check out their websites: www.karmakidsyoga.com and www.yogakids.com.

[15] Jodi Golda Komitor, Founder of Next Generation Yoga offered lion's breath and pose during the Next Generation Yoga Teacher Training too. www.nextgenerationyoga.com. This version is like mine.

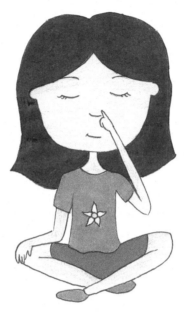

Simple Alternate Nostril Breath

For *nadi shodhana* breath or alternate nostril breathing, I like to do a simplified version for young kids which I learned during the Grounded Kids Yoga Teacher Training.[16]

> With both nostrils, breathe in, breathe out. Press the right index finger onto the right nostril; inhale through the left nostril. With the left index finger, press the left nostril. Remove the right finger. Exhale through the right nostril. Inhale through the right nostril. Press the right nostril with the right index finger. Remove the left index finger from the left nostril. Exhale through the left nostril. Inhale through the left nostril. Continue.

> The breathing exercise can go on for two minutes yet will often end sooner. That's okay. End the breathing exercise when the students begin to stop on their own.

---

[16] www.groundedkids.com. The breath is called Left Breath Right.

Another very valuable breath exercise is in washing machine pose (see Chapter 4 Body Awareness).

Topic

Choose a topic that is familiar to the group so that they can relate to it easily. I like the topic of trees. They are outside year-round, and kids frequently see them. Some class ideas related to trees follow.

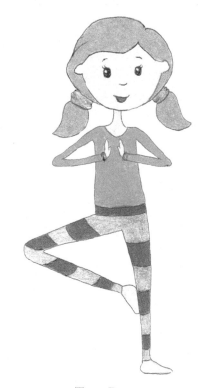

Tree Pose

Trees stand tall and firm, yet their branches are flexible. Your body is strong, and it is also flexible. You need both aspects for balance. Therein lies a simple topic of trees and a dharma talk about balance.

In autumn trees let go of leaves. What are you willing to release? In which ways do you want to let go? Imagine something that is weighing you down. What can you let go of? This is the practice of letting go.

Trees feel the wind, snow, rain, and the feet, knees, and hands of kids climbing on them. They complain about nothing. They are at peace with everything. Let's be like trees. Let's be present. Let's be with what is. Let's neither cling to something nor reject it. This is the practice of nonattachment.

Voice

How do you use your voice? I pause to give words emphasis. After an important concept, I will intentionally pause to give children time to absorb the meaning of what I just said.

I speak softly to grab their attention. Even when they are speaking loudly to each other, one kid hears something soft and listens. Soon others pay attention too.

If the kids are having a day where they cannot keep quiet, I incorporate the voice in their poses.

If I use an unfamiliar word, I'll ask the students if they know its meaning. I'll explain and define it. Later in the class, I'll ask if they can tell me what the word means using their own words. I use these instances as learning opportunities.

There are ways to adjust your voice to enhance learning. Your voice may echo in a small gym. You would need to speak more softly. Kids often pay closer attention when you whisper because listening requires greater focus. When you are in a large gym, your voice may not carry. Then you would project your voice.

Props

I have a few favorite props: *tingshas* and pictures. If the kids are noisy and cannot settle, I may ring tingshas, which are Tibetan bells. When rung softly, they have a very soothing sound that children generally enjoy hearing. I will either ask them to listen to the sound and focus on the duration of time for which they can still hear it, or I'll ask them to keep count of how many times they hear the bell ring. All answers are correct. I simply want them to hear the bell and let the vibration resonate within them. I like to explain to the students at the beginning of class that I may ring these bells if they are making too much noise. That way they associate the ringing with a time to be silent. Sometimes each student wants a turn ringing the bells. This is a wonderful opportunity for them to explore the sound, learn cause and effect, and to feel included. Do they like the sound when it's rung softly or loudly? When you engage the students, they are more likely to cooperate.

I often begin my classes by explaining that yoga is a practice that began over five thousand years ago, in a place called India. People used their bodies to copy the world around them. Thousands of years ago, people saw many animals, trees, and plants around them. For this reason, many of our poses have names of animals, trees, and plants. As time has moved forward, people continued to use their bodies to copy the world around them. Now the world has many inanimate objects. The word *inanimate* describes things that don't breathe.

I have cards with cartoon renditions of animals. For the children, ages five to seven, these cards promote creativity and imagination. These cards promote free expression and movement as children create their own poses. I can shuffle the order of the cards and change the flow of the poses.

Class Arrangement

I enjoy teaching with the yoga mats arranged in a circle. In a circle, each one of us is part of something greater, a big circle. The group shares the energy. Everyone is equal.

Sometimes, however, the movements of other children distract kids. In this instance, I may create two rows facing each other. Now each student has a "partner" for whom he/she is accountable.

Explore how you would like to arrange the room and approach the children. See what works best for you.

Feeling Stuck

If you're feeling stuck, and the creativity just isn't flowing, you may want to implement some of the following practices. You'll know when you are stuck, because the same ideas ceaselessly swirl around in your mind.

I take some time out of my day for me to do something I love. The change of perspective helps to generate new ideas.

I create space in my schedule between the appointments and activities. When I relax and slow down, novel ideas come to me.

I meditate, which creates space between my thoughts and actions. In that space, new concepts form.

At other times, I journal. Maybe all I need is fifteen to twenty minutes. In that time, I explore how I feel by writing all my ideas on paper. I'm decluttering my mind. Seeing my thoughts in writing sometimes enables me to be clear on what I want to say or do.

Part III

Chapter 17

Sample Classes

This chapter offers a sampling of classes to get you started. Each of the following classes illustrate how to put all the components together in a class. You may choose to use these or create your own. I hope you enjoy these and the process of creating a class as much as I do.

Chair Yoga for Ages Eight and Up

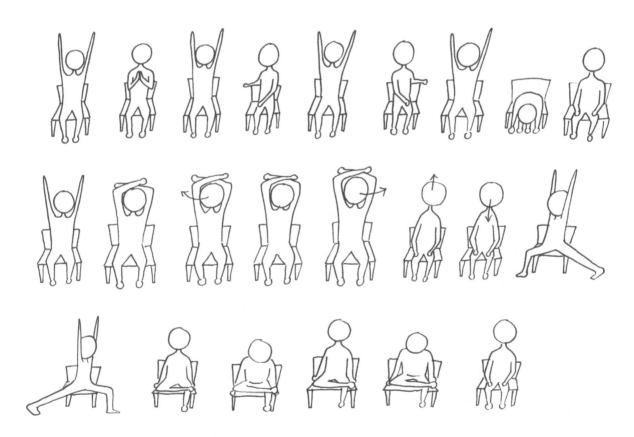

Chair Yoga Sequence

Chair yoga may work well in a classroom setting. It's also ideal for a student with an injury or disability that makes standing a challenge.

Breathe in and raise arms up over head. Breathe out. *Anjali* mudra, bring hands together at the heart. Repeat three times.

Feet rest flat on the ground, parallel like the number eleven. Breathe in, raise arms. Breathe out, twist to the right. The right arm goes behind the chair. The left hand grasps the right knee for resistance. Glance over the right shoulder.

Breathe in, raise arms. Breathe out, twist to the left. The left arm rests on the back of the chair. The right hand grasps the left knee. Gaze over the left shoulder.

Repeat the twists to each side three times.

Breathe in and reach arms up. Breathe out; fold over. Rest tummy on thighs and reach fingers to the toes. Let head dangle. Let frustration, anger, stress, and tension roll off the back.

Breathe in and roll up to seated position. Exhale.

Breathe in. Reach hands and arms up over head. Grasp opposite elbows, making a frame with the arms. Gaze toward the right elbow. Look center. Gaze to the left elbow. Face forward. Release arms and rest hands on lap.

Breathe in while arching the stomach and heart forward. Breathe out while drawing the belly button to the spine and chin to the chest, arching the spine in the opposite direction. Repeat three times.

With the right thigh over the seat, right foot on the ground to the side of the chair, left leg is straight behind you and left foot is on toes, raise hands to the sky, completing seated warrior I on the right side.

Swivel in the chair, with left thigh over the seat, left foot on the ground to the side of the chair. The right leg is straight behind you and right foot is on toes. Raise hands to the sky, completing seated warrior I on the left side.

Turn to face forward.

Place right ankle over left thigh. Breathe out and hinge forward at the hip. Breathe in and sit up. Place left ankle over right thigh. Breathe out and fold forward at the hip. Breathe in and sit up.

If desired, offer two minutes of the chant, "*Sa, ta, na, ma.*" Hand motions are as follows:

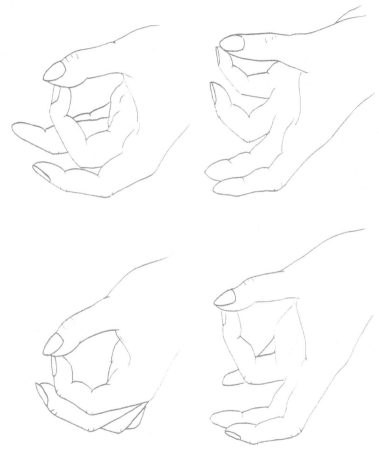

Sa, Ta, Na, Ma

Thumb to index finger.
Thumb to middle finger.
Thumb to ring finger.
Thumb to pinky.

As you move the thumb from finger to finger, say "Sa, ta, na, ma" with each respective finger.[17]

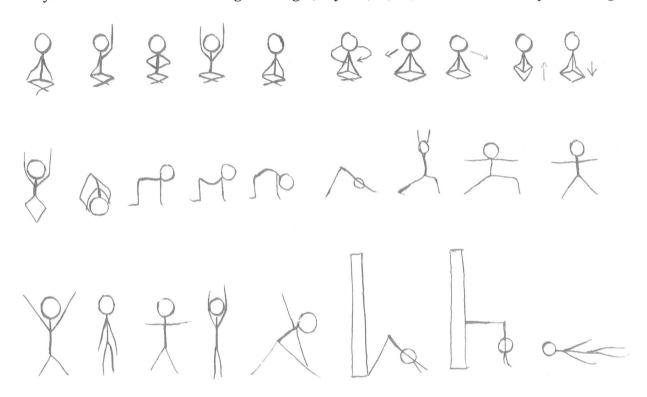

Class on Shapes Sequence (ages three to five)

Class on Shapes for Ages Three to Five

Shapes are all around you. What are your favorite shapes and why? We are going to practice yoga today. While we practice yoga, we are going to notice the shapes our body makes. This class spurs the imagination, gets kids moving, and increases body awareness.

---

[17] Sa Ta Na Ma is used in the Grounded Kids Yoga Teacher Training www.groundedkids.com and in kundalini yoga www.3ho.org?3ho-lifestyle/health-and-healing/kirtan-kriya-sa-ta-na-ma-meditation.

Warm Up

Seated pose (easy pose)

Breathe in and reach up your right arm.
Imagine taking hold of a long string.
Breathe out, pulling down the imaginary string.
Imagine that a big balloon of any shape, size, or color is attached to the string.
Place your pretend balloon on your tummy.
Let's pretend that your tummy is the balloon.

What color is your balloon?
What shape is your balloon?

Place your hands on your tummy, which is the balloon.
Keep your mouth closed, to breathe in and out through your nose.
Breathe in; make the balloon big.
Breathe out; make the balloon small.
Breathe in, big.
Breathe out, small.
That's the way we breathe in yoga, and we'll breathe this way the whole class, in and out through the nose.

Breathe in, reaching up your left arm, and stretch.
If you reach up both arms, your arms make the number eleven.

Let's make circles with our upper bodies.
Please place your hands on your knees, circling the head and torso one way.
Slow the circle down and go in the other direction.

Bend your knees out to the sides and bring the soles of the feet together to be in butterfly pose.
Let's sway side to side like a butterfly.
Now, let's come to stillness.
Next, let's have our knees go up and down.

Let's bring the legs out a little farther, making a diamond shape.
We'll be turtles going into our shells.
Breathe in and reach the arms up.
Breathe out; bring the hands inside the legs, then under the legs.
Fold over as if you were a turtle going into your shell.

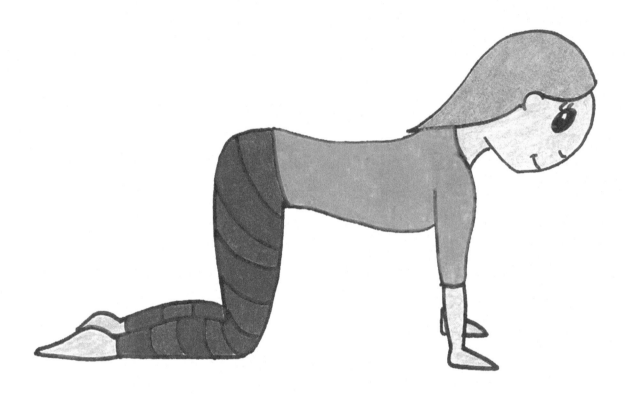

Table Pose

Let's make our bodies look like a rectangle, a tunnel, or a cube.
Please come into table pose.

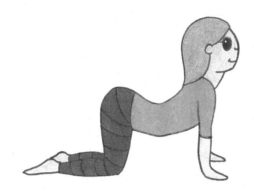

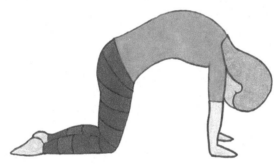

Cow and Cat Pose

Breathe in, cow pose.
Breathe out, cat pose.
Repeat three times and children can say "moo" and "meow" respectively.

Downward-facing dog is a triangle.
Warrior I lunge—arms are the number eleven.
The legs and floor make a four-sided shape.
Warrior II.
Star.
Shining star—breathe in and lift your arms to sixty degrees.
Mountain.

Star.

Moon.

Repeat three times.

These are jumping jacks.[18] They keep us in shape. It's the same word but a different meaning. Our bodies make three shapes to do a jumping jack.

Please come back to star.

Breathe in; breathe out.

Reach your front arm as far forward as you can.

Tap the hand and arm down.

Triangle pose.

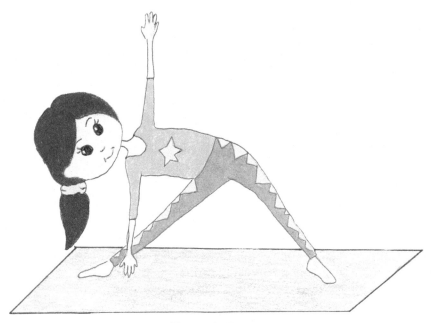

Triangle Pose

How many triangles does your body make in this pose? Let's count.

Triangle pose on the other side.

---

[18] I learned to combine these three poses to create a jumping jack during Next Generation Yoga Teacher Training with Founder Jodi Golda Komitor. www.generationyoga.com

We play a game that utilizes shapes. There are many available; simply go to your local toy store. Playing a game during a yoga class allows the children to be silly and spontaneous. Silliness and spontaneity spur creativity, imagination, and happiness.

Do sun salutations (see Chapter 6 Letting Go) to give thanks for this day.

Please come to the wall and do these poses:

- Downward-facing dog
- L-shape with legs on the wall
- Seated staff pose is also an L
- Relaxation pose.

The reading is from *Starbright: Meditations for Children,* which is listed in the last chapter of this book.

I modify a reading about clouds. I mention various shapes that the clouds make in the sky.

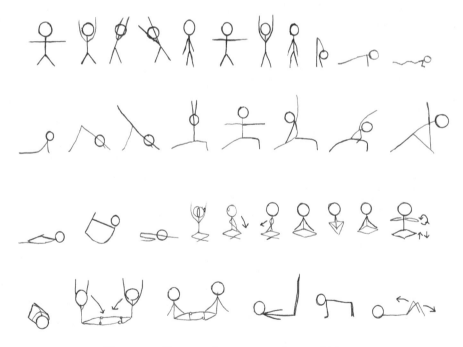

Class on Shapes Sequence (ages 5-7)

Class on Shapes for Ages Five to Seven

I tell the children that the class is about the words *shape* and *shapes*. We keep our bodies in shape. Our bodies have a shape. What are the shapes we can make with our bodies during our yoga practice? The educational purposes of this class are to gain body awareness, learn how to take care of the body through exercise and breathing, and to learn shapes.

Set up the mats in a circle.
As a warm-up, have the kids do sun salutations.
Who feels stretched, stronger, calm, energized?
Sun salutations do all of this to us. They keep us in shape.

With the kids still standing, have them come into star pose. They are stars. Let them be shining stars. You may want to introduce an affirmation. Breathe in, raise your arms, and be a shining star. Exhale and say, "I like being me!"

Star pose. Now your body is the shape of a star. Notice that your hands touch your neighbors' hands. The sides of your feet touch your neighbors'. You and your neighbors' arms and legs make the shape of a diamond!

Inhale, arms overhead, interlacing fingers. Lean to the right. Crescent moon shape.
Exhale, lean to the left.

Mountain, star, moon. These three shapes make a jumping jack.

Mountain pose. Stand tall. Exhale. Hand to foot pose. Inhale. Plank. Exhale *chaturanga* or low plank. Inhale. Cobra. Exhale. Downward-facing dog. This is a triangle.

Inhale; lift right leg. Place the right foot between the hands. Warrior I lunge. Place your heel on the floor. Warrior I.

Warrior II. Our legs with the floor, make a four-sided shape. Inhale, peaceful warrior. Exhale, side angle stretch.

Come into a triangle pose. How many triangles is your body making now? Let's count.

Plank. The body with the floor makes a rectangle. Chaturanga, cobra. Now your back is a semi-circle. Downward-facing Dog. We are making a triangle again.

Inhale; please lift the left leg. Place the left foot between your hands. Warrior I lunge to a warrior I. We've made a four-sided shape with our left leg and the floor. What other shapes have four sides?

Inhale to peaceful warrior; exhale to side angle stretch. Now let's explore triangle pose on the left side.

Let's come down to the floor on our bellies. Hold onto the right ankle with the right hand to get a big stretch in your quadricep. This is the muscle in the front of the thigh. Stretching it helps us stay flexible. Strengthening it and stretching it keeps us in shape.

Hold onto the left ankle with the left hand to get a big stretch in the quadricep of your left leg. Now we are staying in balance because what we do on one side of the body, we also do on the other.

Please hold onto both ankles. Imagine stretching your knees toward the back of the room. Inhale; please lift the heart and thighs. Press the ankles into the hands and the hands into the ankles. You are now in a bow shape!

Child's pose.

Easy pose. Your legs are crossed in this seated pose. Inhale and put your arms up to the sky. Your arms look like the number eleven. Exhale and twist. Your left hand is on the right knee. The right hand is behind you. Inhale, letting the arms float up on the breath. Exhale, twisting to the left. The right hand goes on the left knee. The left hand goes directly behind the back. Repeat two more times. We have been twisting. A twist is a shape.

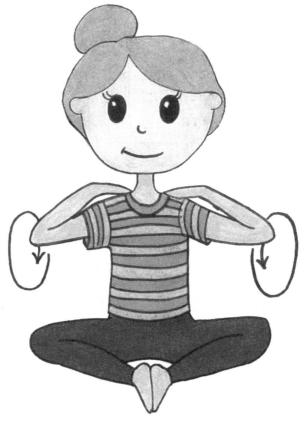

Butterfly Pose

Butterfly. Rock side to side in butterfly. Bring the body to stillness. Then, please move the knees up and down. Let's add the upper wings, bringing the hands to the shoulders. The four fingers are in front. The thumb is behind. Now the upper wings go in circles. The lower wings go up and down.

Let's make a diamond with our legs.

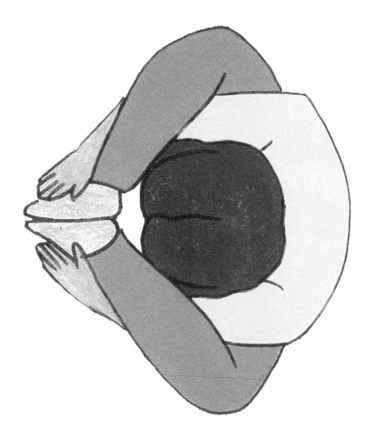

Turtle Pose[19]

Turtle pose. Inhale and put your arms up to the sky. Your arms look like the number eleven. Exhale and lower your arms so that your hands go inside and under your legs. Your back is a semicircle, like the shell of a turtle.

Lying on your back, please lift your legs and feet up to the sky. You are making the letter L with your body.

---

[19] Yoga Pretzels by Tara Guber and Leah Kalish

Bridge pose. This is another semicircle.

Please bring your feet to the outer reaches of the mat. Sway the knees side to side as if they were windshield wipers.

I may bring the children to the wall and offer the same poses I did for the children ages three to five.

I offer the same reading about clouds at the end of class.

Class on Shapes for Ages Eight to Ten

I tell the children that the class is about the words *shape* and *shapes*. We keep our bodies in shape. We stay in shape by exercising and eating healthfully. What does it mean to eat healthfully? We can drink water instead of soda for example.

Let's close our eyes and focus on the breath now. Notice the breath as it goes in and out of the body. Inhaling deeply and exhaling completely in this circular rhythm enables the body to stay healthy and alive. *We breathe approximately twenty thousand breaths in a day.*[20] Each breath brings oxygen and nutrients from food to every cell in the body. We stay in shape by exercising and eating healthfully. What kind of exercise do you enjoy?

Our bodies have a shape. What are the shapes we can make with our bodies during our yoga practice? The educational purposes of this class are to gain body awareness, learn how to take care of the body through exercise and breathing, and to learn shapes.

Set up the mats in a circle.

As a warm-up, have the kids do sun salutations.

Who feels stretched, stronger, calm, energized?

Sun salutations do all of this to us. They keep us in shape.

---

[20] http://www.lung.org/your-lungs/

With the kids still standing, have them come into star pose. They are stars. Let them be shining stars. You may want to introduce an affirmation. Breathe in, raise your arms, and be a shining star. Exhale and say, "I like being me!"

Star pose. Now your body is the shape of a star. Notice that your hands touch your neighbors' hands. The sides of your feet touch your neighbors'. You and your neighbors' arms and legs make the shape of a diamond!

Inhale, arms overhead, interlacing fingers. Lean to the right. Crescent moon shape. Exhale, lean to the left.

Mountain, star, moon. These three shapes make a jumping jack.

Mountain pose. Stand tall. Exhale. Hand to foot pose. Inhale. Plank. Exhale *chaturanga* or low plank. Inhale. Cobra. Exhale. Downward-facing dog. This is a triangle.

Inhale; lift right leg. Place the right foot between the hands. Warrior I lunge. Place your heel on the floor. Warrior I.

Warrior II. Our legs with the floor, make a quadrilateral. Inhale, peaceful warrior. Exhale, side angle stretch.

Come into a triangle pose. How many triangles is your body making now? Let's count.

Do you know what a triangle with two equal sides is called? It's called an isosceles triangle.

Plank. The body with the floor makes a rectangle. Chaturanga, cobra. Now your back is a semicircle. Downward-facing Dog. We are making a triangle again.

Inhale; please lift the left leg. Place the left foot between your hands. Warrior I lunge to a warrior I. We've made a quadrilateral or a quadrangle with our left leg and the floor. What other shapes are quadrilaterals?

Inhale to peaceful warrior; exhale to side angle stretch. Now let's explore triangle pose on the left side.

Let's come down to the floor on our bellies. Hold onto the right ankle with the right hand to get a big stretch in your quadricep. This is the muscle in the front of the thigh. Stretching it helps us stay flexible. Strengthening it and stretching it keeps us in shape.

Hold onto the left ankle with the left hand to get a big stretch in the quadricep of your left leg. Now we are staying in balance because what we do on one side of the body, we also do on the other.

Please hold onto both ankles. Imagine stretching your knees toward the back of the room. Inhale; please lift the heart and thighs. Press the ankles into the hands and the hands into the ankles. You are now in a bow shape!

Child's pose.

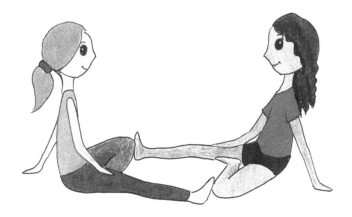

Rectangle Pose

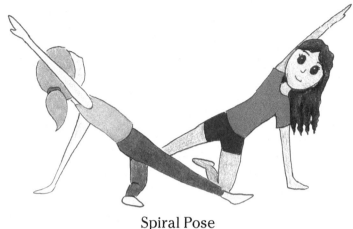

Spiral Pose

Find a friend and partner up. Place the legs in partner *janusirsasana* (rectangle pose), so that when the kids face one another the perimeter of their legs makes a rectangle. I tell them to make the number four shape with their legs. One foot should touch their partner's knee. Inhale, arms up. Exhale, fold over the extended leg. Inhale, cartwheel an arm behind you to come into inclined plane. Now you and your friend together have made a spiral. A spiral is a type of twist.

Butterfly. Rock side to side in butterfly. Bring the body to stillness. Then, please move the knees up and down. Let's add the upper wings, bringing the hands to the shoulders. The four fingers are in front. The thumb is behind. Now the upper wings go in circles. The lower wings go up and down.

Let's make a diamond with our legs.

Turtle pose. Inhale and put your arms up to the sky. Your arms look like the number eleven. Exhale and lower your arms so that your hands go inside and under your legs. Your back is a semicircle, like the shell of a turtle.

Lying on your back, please lift your legs and feet up to the sky. You are making the letter L with your body.

Bridge pose. This is another semicircle.

Please bring your feet to the outer reaches of the mat. Sway the knees side to side as if they were windshield wipers.

I may bring the children to the wall and offer the same poses I did for the children ages three to five.

I offer the same reading about clouds at the end of class.

Animals Breathe, So Do We for Ages Three to Five

People breathe, and so do animals. Chairs, tables, and other objects that are not living cannot breathe.

You are always breathing. While practicing yoga, focus on how you breathe. Please keep your mouth closed, to breathe in and out through the nose. The educational purpose of this class is to gain breath and body awareness.

Please place your hand on your tummy. Breathe in through the nose and feel the cool air come in. Breathe out through the nose, and feel the warm air go out.

Breathe in deeply, and with your hand on your tummy, feel the tummy rise. Breathe out, and feel the tummy go down.

Frog pose is next. This is not a frog that jumps. This frog will stretch. Squat. Hands are on the floor. Breathe in and lift the hips. Breathe out while you lower the hips and lift your face. Repeat this sequence at least three times.

Easy pose. What sound does a frog make? Encourage the children to breathe in deeply then repeat "ribbit" several times.

Have the children stand in mountain pose. Stand strong and stable like a mountain. Ask what gorillas eat. They eat bananas and coconuts.

Come to star pose with bent knees (this is your gorilla).[21] Breathe in; reach the arms up to the banana trees to get two bananas. With two fists, gently tap the middle of the chest while saying, "Bananaaas."

Have them do a similar stretch next, this time reaching both hands to the right to grasp a coconut. Gently place it on the ground. Breathe in; reach for a coconut with both arms to the left. Breathe out as you place the coconut by your left foot. Breathe in deeply in shining star pose. Exhale while both fists gently tap the middle of the chest and the children softly call out, "Coconuts!"

Table pose. Breathe in then say "moo," in cow pose as you breathe out. Breathe in. Say, "meow," in cat pose as you breathe out.

Come up on the knees. Breathe in. Take out your lion's paws. Stick out your tongue and exhale a soft lion roar. Repeat this cycle three times as well. If I'm in a classroom, I have the kids "roar" softly. If we are in a gym or outdoor space, I permit the kids to roar loudly.

Butterfly, rocking and moving knees up and down.

Turtle pose.

A turtle goes into its shell to feel safe, cozy, peaceful and protected.

Whether they are laying down in *savasana* which is Sanskrit for relaxation pose, or sitting upright, I have them massage one finger on their forehead. Imagine that your forehead is a screen and you are wiping the dust off it. On your screen, imagine where you go to feel safe, cozy, peaceful and protected.

I end with a meditation or an affirmation about kindness. There are many books with meditations or affirmations that you can use, or you can make up your own.

---

[21] Gorilla is a goddess pose, but I don't call it goddess pose because often I work at schools and don't want to say anything with a religious connotation. I will recommend a star pose with bent knees.

Animals Breathe, So Do We for Ages Five to Seven

People breathe and so do animals. Chairs, tables, and other objects that are not living do not breathe. The educational purpose of this class is to gain breath and body awareness.

We are always breathing. While practicing yoga, we focus on how we breathe. We pay attention to how it feels to breathe. Let's practice. Please keep your mouth closed, to breathe in and out through the nose.

Please place your hand on your tummy. Breathe in through the nose and feel the cool air come in. Breathe out through the nose, feel the warm air go out.

Breathe in deeply, and with your hand on your tummy, feel the tummy rise.

Frog pose is next. This is not a frog that jumps. This frog will stretch. Squat. Hands are on the floor. Breathe in and lift the hips. Breathe out while you lower the hips and lift your face. Repeat this sequence at least three times.

End with the squat and have the frog "take an elevator" to stand. (Stand up after squatting in frog pose).

Place your fingers gently on your throat and say, "Ribbit." What do you feel? The answer is a vibration.

Mountain pose. Gorillas eat bananas and coconuts.

Come to star pose with bent knees (this is your gorilla pose). Breathe in; reach the arms up to the banana trees to get two bananas. With two fists, gently tap the middle of the chest while saying, "Bananaaas."

Come back to star pose. Turn to the right, transforming the pose into a warrior I lunge. With hands reaching up, inhale and imagine you are reaching for a coconut from the coconut tree. Exhale; bring the coconut to the inside of the right foot. Inhale; swing the coconut to the left foot. Exhale, and bring it back to right foot. Inhale; swing the coconut overhead to the left foot. Exhale; bring the coconut one final time to the right foot, and gently place it on the ground.[22]

Star pose. Breath in and raise arms to the left to reach for the imaginary coconut from another tree. Exhale, and please lower the coconut to the left foot. Inhale and swing it to the right foot. Exhale, and bring it to the left foot. Inhale, lift the coconut overhead, and then place the coconut by the right foot. Exhale, gently place it by the left foot. Breathe in deeply, standing in shining star pose. Exhale while both fists gently tap the middle of the chest and the children softly call out, "Coconuts!"

How do you feel after you say coconuts or bananas? Some possible answers are silly or happy.

These are positive feelings. When you say positive, happy words, you feel better. The good news is that you can choose the words you want to say.

Let's give thanks for this day by doing three sun salutations. Play a song about enjoying sunshine. There are many available on music apps. Speak about how the body needs sunshine, water and air to live.

Are you feeling hot now? Let's do cooling breath. Curl the tongue and sip in air as if your tongue were a straw. Exhale through the nose. This breath cools you when you are feeling hot and calms you when you are feeling angry. Not everyone can curl his or her tongue. Alternatively, a student can place the tongue on the roof of the mouth behind the two front teeth while breathing in through the mouth.

Cow and Cat Poses. Children can say "moo" and "meow" respectively. Repeat three times.

Come up on to the knees. Breathe in. Take out your lion's paws. Stick out your tongue and exhale a soft lion roar. Repeat this cycle, three times as well. If I'm in a classroom, I have the kids "roar" softly. If we are in a gym or outdoor space, I permit the kids to roar loudly.

Butterfly, rocking and moving knees up and down.

Turtle pose.

---

[22] Yoga Pretzels by Tara Guber and Leah Kalish. In this gorilla pose, students sway in a different manner and state affirmations.

A turtle goes into its shell to feel safe, cozy, peaceful and protected.[23]

Whether they are laying down in *savasana* or relaxation pose, or sitting upright, I have them massage one finger on their foreheads. Imagine that your forehead is a screen and you are wiping the dust off it.[24] On your screen, imagine where you go to feel safe, cozy, peaceful and protected.

I end with a meditation or an affirmation about kindness. There are many books with meditations or affirmations that you can use, or you can make up your own.

Animals Breathe, So Do We for Ages Eight to Ten

You are always breathing. While practicing yoga, focus on how you breathe. *People breathe approximately twenty thousand breaths in a day.*[25] The breath brings oxygen and nutrients from food to every cell in the body. Breathing fully helps you feel more alive. Please close your eyes to bring your attention inside your body. Bringing your awareness inward will give you information about your body so you can take the best care of it.

Breathe in through the nose and feel the cool air come in. Breathe out through the nose, and feel the warm air go out.

Please place one hand on your stomach and the other on your chest. Breathe in deeply and feel the breath travel from your nasal passageway, down your throat, all the way down to your stomach. Breathe out, and feel the belly soften.

I will then ask the students to come to standing. Frog pose is next. This is not a frog that jumps. This frog will stretch. Squat. Hands are on the floor. Breathe in and lift the hips. Breathe out while you lower the hips and lift your face. Repeat this sequence at least three times.

End with the squat and have the frog "take an elevator" to stand. (Stand up after squatting in frog pose).

---

[23] Yoga Pretzels by Tara Guber and Leah Kalish. In this turtle pose, students say a different affirmation about protection.

[24] Christine McArdle-Oquendo offers a screen meditation for kids. www.christinemcardleoquendo.com

[25] http://www.lung.org/your-lungs/

Place your fingers gently on your throat and say, "Ribbit." What do you feel? The answer is a vibration. What is a vibration? A vibration is energy. Each word has energy or a vibration.

Mountain pose.

Gorillas eat bananas and coconuts.

Star pose with bent knees (this is your gorilla pose). Breathe in and reach the arms up to the banana trees to get two bananas. With two fists, gently tap the sternum of the chest while saying, "Bananaaas." The sternum is the bone located in the center of the chest.

Star pose. Turn to the right, transforming the pose into a warrior I lunge. With hands reaching up, inhale and imagine you are reaching for a coconut from the coconut tree. Exhale; bring the coconut to the inside of the right foot. Inhale and swing the coconut to the left foot. Exhale, and bring it back to right foot. Inhale and swing the coconut overhead to the left foot. Exhale and bring the coconut one final time to the right foot and gently, place it on the ground.

Star pose. Breathe in and swivel arms to the left to reach for the imaginary coconut from another tree. Exhale; please lower the coconut to the left foot. Inhale and swing it to the right foot. Exhale; bring it to the left foot. Inhale, lift the coconut overhead and then place the coconut by the right foot. Exhale; gently place it by your left foot. Breathe in deeply in shining star pose. Exhale while both fists gently tap the sternum and the children softly call out, "Coconuts!"

I mentioned earlier that when we speak, a vibration is created inside the body. How do you feel after you say coconuts or bananas? Some possible answers are silly or happy.

These are positive feelings. When we say positive, happy words, a positive vibration is created in the body and we feel better. If we say hostile, insulting words, a negative vibration is created in the body and we feel worse. The good news is that we can choose the words we want to say. In that way, we have control over whether we are creating a negative or positive vibration in the body.

Let's give thanks for this day by doing three sun salutations. Speak about how the body needs sunshine, water, and air to live.

Are you feeling hot now? Let's do a cooling breath. Curl the tongue and sip in air as if your tongue were a straw. If your tongue does not curl, please place it on the roof of the mouth behind the two front teeth and breathe in through the mouth. Exhale through the nose. This breath cools you when you are feeling hot and calms you when you are feeling angry.

Table pose. Breathe in, dipping the stomach down and lifting the chin, in cow pose. Breathe out, arching the spine up and tucking the chin, in cat pose. Repeat three times.

Come up on to the knees. Breathe in. Take out your lion's paws. Stick out your tongue and exhale a soft lion roar. Repeat these steps three times as well. If I'm in a classroom, I have the kids "roar" softly. If we are in a gym or outdoor space, I permit the kids to roar loudly.

Butterfly, rocking and moving knees up and down.

Turtle pose.

A turtle goes into its shell to feel safe, cozy, peaceful and protected.

Whether they are laying down on the back in *savasana* or relaxation pose, or sitting upright, I have them massage one finger on their forehead. Imagine that your forehead is a screen and you are wiping the dust off it. On your screen, imagine where you go to feel safe, cozy, peaceful and protected.

I end with a meditation or an affirmation about kindness. There are many books with meditations or affirmations that you can use, or you can make up your own.

For this age group, I may also read the following. It's the Sanskrit chant, "*Lokah samastah sukhino bhavantu,*" translated to English.

May all beings be happy and free.

And may the thoughts, words, and actions of my own life contribute, in some way, to the happiness and freedom for all.

I come up with an idea and consider how I could explain this topic to a very young child. I break the topic down into bite-size pieces that a small child could grasp. Let me now take you through some of my thought processes regarding a yoga class for children on the *niyama saucha*.

Class on the Niyama Saucha

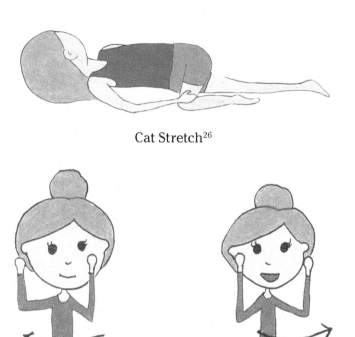

Cat Stretch[26]

Examples of Twist Poses

One of the basic principles of yoga is *saucha,* which means cleanliness. When we think of clean, what comes to mind? I like to ask an open-ended question after I've introduced the topic to properly

---

[26] The cat stretch pose I use has the far arm down alongside the body. In Kundalini Yoga, the far arm is facing up overhead. https://www.3ho.org/3ho-lifestyle/daily-routine/sleep/wake-routine

gauge the student's knowledge base. I include lots of twists to cleanse the body. Included in a yoga class on cleanliness is the following educational information:

- Eating a healthy diet to avoid putting toxins in the body.
- Benefits of drinking water to keep the kidneys functioning properly and rid the body of toxins.
- Germs: bacterium and viruses. What are they? How are they treated? What does the body do to fight them off?

Kids love to learn about their bodies, and children ages eight and up will eat up this information.

For children ages seven and under, I may have a class about feeling good and thinking clearly.

- What kinds of food make us feel good?
- Fruits and vegetables. Their bright colors mean that they have vitamins and minerals, which make us strong and energized.
- Junk food. I acknowledge that they like it, but what happens if you eat too much of it?
- Which habits or activities help you think clearly?
- During which games and activities do you feel happy and strong?
- Let's explore poses that help us feel this way.

For the very young children, ages three to five, I may share this poem:

Fuzzy Wuzzy was a bear.
Fuzzy Wuzzy had no hair.
Fuzzy Wuzzy wasn't fuzzy.
Was he?[27]

- I will explain that fuzzy may mean hairy. It can also mean cloudy thinking.
- How do we think in a way that is not cloudy? We take care of our bodies.
- I will approach the topic of saucha without calling it saucha.
- My class on shapes is one example of a saucha class.

---

[27] Rudyard Kipling (public domain 1892)

Alternate Nostril Breathing

Warrior poses: warrior I and warrior II. In warrior II, hold *gyan mudra*, thumb to index finger. This mudra relaxes the body and focuses the mind. Explain to preschoolers that they are looking through the hole the fingers make.

Stand firmly on your feet, feeling strong and majestic like a mountain.

Stretching frog pose. Squat. Breathe in as hips rise; keep your hands on the floor near your toes. Breathe out as hips lower and head rises. Please repeat at least three times.

Eagle pose. Maybe keep toes of wrapped foot on the ground for support. Criss-cross elbows. Describe the eagle's ability to see the big picture on top of a mountain or clifftop. Be like an eagle, noticing the world around you.

Consider all the ways you can take good care of yourself: good nutrition, exercise, breathing, and pausing. Can you think of other examples of good health practices?

Class on Satya or Truth

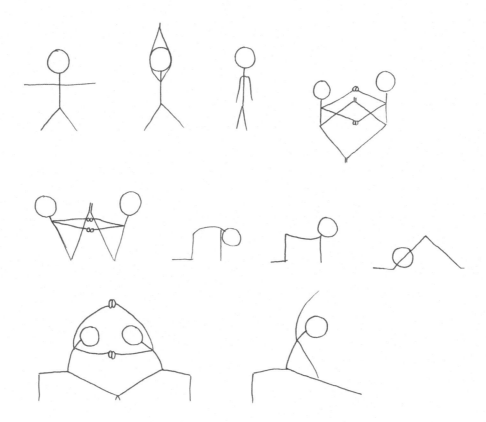

Satya Class Sequence (ages Eight to Ten)

You may want to begin class with a discussion of what it means to be true to yourself, to speak your own truth. There are many children's books on the topic. If you choose, you may start by reading a short picture book on the topic.

How do you express yourself when you are angry? Do you yell? How do you feel when someone yells at you?

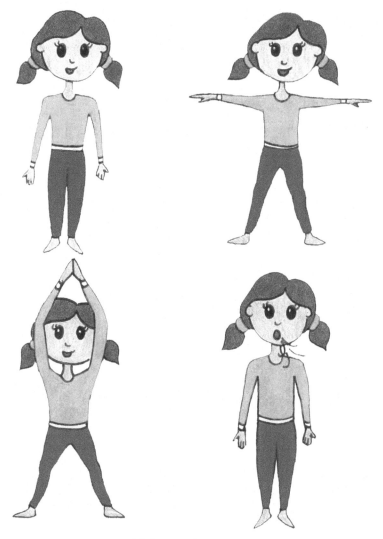

Volcano Pose

Volcano Breath:[28] Breathe in; jump to a star pose. Breathe in; keep legs apart, jump, and bring palms together overhead. Now you are an upside-down V-shape. Breathe out through the mouth with a loud noise while you jump into mountain pose. This is your volcano erupting.

---

[28] YogaKids offers volcano pose and volcano breath. http://yogakids.com/

A quiet voice inside guides you. To hear it, breathe and listen.

Sun salutations.

Every time you speak your truth, you build your self-respect.

"I love being me!" Give yourself a hug.

Seated straddle partner pose (see-saw)[29, 30]. Hold hands and lean back and forth.

For younger kids, straddle stretch. Make legs look like the letter V.

Partner Boat pose[31] (ages 8 to 10, press feet together and hold hands). The younger kids (ages 5 to 7) can explore boat pose individually.

Cat/cow.

Dolphin.

Warrior II partner pose—outer edge of back foot touches your partner's outer edge of foot.

In partner warrior II, see if you can arch back to touch your partner's hands in the air.

Warrior twist. For the younger kids, peaceful warrior.

I suggest sharing inspirational quotes by Joseph Campbell.

Class on Man-Made Objects

During the practice of yoga, people use their bodies to imitate their surroundings. With time, the environment contained more man-made objects. Let's explore these objects. The educational purpose of this class is for the student to gain body awareness and to experience his/her connection to the global community.

Washing machine pose.

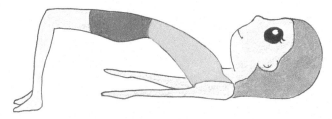

Bridge Pose

---

[29] Marsha Wenig, founder of YogaKids International, http://yogakids.com

[30] Yoga Pretzels by Tara Guber and Leah Kalish

[31] Yoga Pretzels by Tara Guber and Leah Kalish

Navasana—boat pose (sing "Row, Row Your Boat"[32] with the preschoolers).

Taking a boat from one location to another connects people from different lands or islands. You get to see more people.

Bridge pose.

Car pose.[33, 34]

Bridges and cars also bring people together.

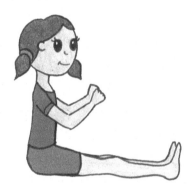

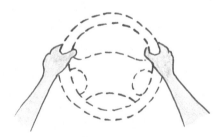

Car Pose

---

[32] The tune with the lyrics was recorded in 1881 by Eliphalet Oram Lyte.

[33] Shari Vilchez-Blatt of Karma Kids Yoga offered a teacher training in which I learned this car pose, see saw, and partner boat pose as well as many other transportation poses to capture a young child's imagination.

[34] Jodi Golda Komitor, Founder of Next Generation Yoga, also taught a very playful car pose. www.nextgenerationyoga.com

Airplane pose (warrior III).

Airplanes connect people and cultures. In some ways, the world becomes a smaller place because we can go far distances quickly. In other ways, the world becomes a bigger place, because we have the means to travel a far distance to connect with people.

How do we connect with people in our town?

Table pose.

Chair pose.

One friend can be the chair; another can be the table. Kids can group together with multiple chairs and tables to share conversation.

Train pose. (Stand and march). Breathe out, "Choo, choo!"

During relaxation, I offer a meditation in which I speak about the love in your heart. Feel it travel throughout your body (specify body parts). Let that love shine out to the room. Send that love to someone you love who is not here in this room. Notice how love connects us to others in the world around us. This love is ever present in your hearts. Feel this love throughout your day.

Chapter 18

How To Practice Yoga Off The Mat

To be a valued kids' yoga instructor, I find it's not enough to know the benefits. I find it necessary to look deep inside myself and ask, "Why do I do this?"

I grew up in the 1970s. While life seemed simpler than it is today, I struggled a lot with inner turmoil as a child. I lacked the skills to cope with certain challenges and overcome many obstacles. As a yoga instructor, I teach the skills I now possess, to a younger generation.

During my youth, when I had a problem, I'd obsess about it. I assumed I needed to focus on the problem to come up with a solution. Sometimes I'd ruminate over an obstacle, come up with various solutions, and choose one. In theory, nothing is wrong with this. I was quite self-reliant at a very young age. Yet, I wasn't happy. Pouring all my effort into scrutinizing what wasn't working in my life clearly brought me down. My thoughts were negative. I was moody and depressed.

I thought criticism was normal. I thought criticizing someone was a way of helping. Pointing out what was wrong seemed like a constructive way to help a person improve.

I've come a long way in elevating my thought processes. While I can follow the logic of my former perspective, I now have a very different approach. I no longer ignore problems. I know they exist. I'm just open to the possibility of something else. It's as if I were holding a problem in my hand. My younger self would have squeezed my hand around the problem. The only thing my hand was holding was the problem. Plus, my hand became a fist. I was angry.

Today, I still hold problems in my hands, but I keep my palms facing up, fingers unclenched. My hands are outreached, ready to receive something positive: sunshine to melt the problems or water to wash them away. Of course, the hand is simply a metaphor for how I now approach challenges in my life. I'm aware of the problem, yet my heart and mind remain open to receive. Maybe someone's kindness or suggestion provides a solution. Maybe laughter helps assuage pain. Perhaps all I need to do is replace a negative thought with a positive one.

As a child, I was criticized by adults who thought they were helping me. Instead, their negative words pulled me down. Today, I teach children to choose the positive ones. They're uplifting.

Here's an exercise I enjoy doing, and I encourage students to do the same.

> Begin by observing your thoughts. Use an open-minded approach. Don't judge the thoughts you are having. This may be easier said than done because you may find yourself judging your own thoughts, and that's okay. Simply observe where your thoughts are. Remember my analogy with the picnic blanket. Reject nothing. Simply notice.

When you hear a negative thought, isolate it. Next, ask yourself, "How can I phrase this comment in a more neutral way? Can I rewrite this thought in a positive form? Notice with each revision how your body relaxes, and you cheer up.

Another worthwhile exercise is to keep a gratitude journal. The practice of regularly expressing your gratitude in writing helps train the mind to think in positive ways. In Sanskrit we call these ingrained thought patterns of the mind *samskaras*. They are the thought-processing patterns of the mind. The practice of yoga asana, chanting, meditation, pranayama, and positive thinking help change these paths, tracks, or patterns to higher elevations. The higher self, alternatively known as the neutral mind, guides us into a calmer, more peaceful space.

I love the following Buddhist meditation.

> Watch your thoughts; they become your words.
>
> Watch your words; they become your actions.
>
> Watch your actions; they become your habits.
>
> Watch your habits; they become your character.
>
> Watch your character; it becomes your destiny.

Chapter 19
Suggested Reading

These books are among my favorites for meditations, ideas for classes, and self-help. The children's book entitled *A Bad Case of Stripes* made the list because the story is about a girl who learns how to speak her truth. It's an excellent book upon which to base a class.

Garth, Maureen. *Moonbeams: A Collection of Children's Meditations.* New York, New York: HarperCollins Publisher, 1992.

Garth, Maureen. *Starbright: A Collection of Children's Meditations.* New York, New York: HarperCollins Publisher, 1991.

Jenkins, PhD. Peggy J. *Nurturing Spirituality in Children.* Hillsboro, Oregon: Beyond Words Publishing Inc., 1995.

Maureen Murdock, Maureen. *Spinning Inward: Using Guided Imagery with Children for Learning, Creativity and Relaxation.* Boston, Massachusetts: Shambhala Publishing, 1987.

Shannon, David. *A Bad Case of Stripes.* New York, New York: The Blue Sky Press, 1998.

Tolle, Eckhart. *The Power of Now.* Vancouver B.C., Canada: Namaste Publishing, and Novato, California: New World Library, 2004.

About the Author

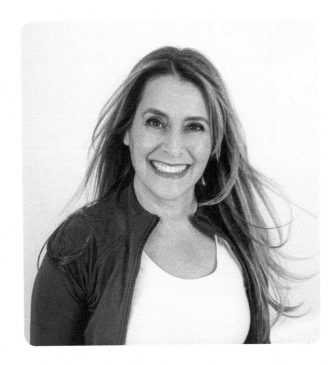

Stacey Pinke has always had a passion for writing and is very excited about the publication of her first book! As a Registered Yoga Teacher and Dietitian, Stacey inspires and encourages people to be the best version of themselves. She has over ten years of experience teaching yoga to children in New Jersey public schools and community centers. When she is not working, Stacey is a mom who enjoys reading, hiking, and spending time with family. Please visit her website www.yoga-blossoms.com to find out more about Yoga Blossoms Kids Yoga Teacher Training, workshops and other services.

About the Illustrator

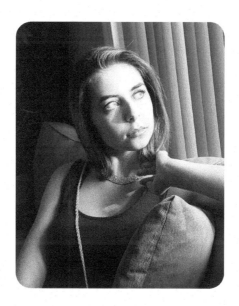

With gratitude and pride, Maria Gronowska is thrilled to have made her first professional artistic contribution. Having been interested in art since age nine, she created the illustrations for this book at age fourteen. Maria is currently enrolled in a university in France to study art.

References

Cameron, Julia. *The Artist's Way: A Spiritual Path to Higher Creativity.* Los Angeles, CA: Jeremy P. Tarcher/Perigee, 1992. Print.

Emoto, Masaru. *The Hidden Messages in Water.* Hillsboro, Or.: Beyond Words Pub., 2004. Print.

Vilchez-Blatt, Shari. "Yoga Poses." *Karma Kids Yoga: Teacher Training Course Manual.* N.p.: n.p., 2008. 11, 25, 43, 51, 60. Print.

Jenkins, Peggy Davison., and Peggy Davison. Jenkins. "Chapter 11: Watch Your Words." *Nurturing Spirituality in Children: Simple Hands-on Activities.* Hillsboro, Or.: Beyond Words Pub., 1995. N. pag. Print.

Komitor, Jodi. *Next Generation Yoga: Why Kids Love Yoga! NGY Teacher Training for 2-7 year olds.* By Jodi B Komitor MA, RYT. 2008. Print.

Rodriguera, Chara, and Richard Gange. "Chara." *Chara RSS.* Roman Media, n.d. Web. 17 Feb. 2015. <http://chara.tv/>. Life Programs

Wenig, Marsha. *YogaKids: Educating the Whole Child Through Yoga.* New York, NJ: Stewart, Tabori & Chang, 2003. Print.

Wilson, Erin and Shari Vilchez-Blatt. "The Power of Positive Thinking." *Karma Kids Yoga: Teen Yoga Teacher Training Course Manual.* N.p.:n.p., 2010. 121.Print.